Functional Progressions for Sport Rehabilitation

Steven R. Tippett, MS, PT, SCS, ATC
Great Plains Sports Medicine and Rehabilitation Center
Peoria, IL

Michael L. Voight, MED, PT, SCS, OCS, ATC
Berkshire Institute of Orthopaedic and Sports Physical Therapy
Wyomissing, PA

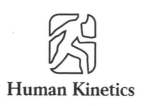

Human Kinetics

Library of Congress Cataloging-in-Publication Data

Tippett, Steven R., 1956-
  Functional progressions for sport rehabilitation / Steven R.
Tippett, Michael L. Voight.
    p.   cm.
  Includes bibliographical references and index.
  ISBN 0-87322-660-7
  1. Sports injuries--Patients--Rehabilitation.   2. Sports physical
therapy. I. Voight, Michael L., 1959- . II. Title.
RT97.T53   1995
617.1'027--dc20   93-46409
                                                                                            CIP

ISBN: 0-87322-660-7

Developmental Editor: Mary E. Fowler; **Assistant Editors:** Ed Giles, Jacqueline Blakley, Henry Woolsey, and Karen Bojda; **Copyeditor:** John Wentworth; **Proofreader:** Karen Dorman; **Indexer:** Barbara E. Cohen; **Typesetters and Layout Artists:** Ruby Zimmerman and Kathy Boudreau-Fuoss; **Text Design:** Jody Boles; **Cover Designer:** Jack Davis; **Photographer (cover & interior):** Karen Maier; **Illustrators:** Tom Janowski and Craig Ronto; **Printer:** United Graphics; **Models:** Ed Becker, Mark Corsentino, Lynette Davis, Chris Gensler, Brian McGrath, Melissa Neuhalfen, J.D. Nimrick, Mark Norman, Lance A. Reiman, Erin Schmitt, Dan Troy.

Printed in the United States of America   10 9 8 7 6 5 4 3 2 1

Human Kinetics
P.O. Box 5076, Champaign, IL 61825-5076
1-800-747-4457

Canada: Human Kinetics, Box 24040, Windsor, ON N8Y 4Y9
1-800-465-7301 (in Canada only)

Europe: Human Kinetics, P.O. Box IW14, Leeds LS16 6TR, England
(44) 532 781708

Australia: Human Kinetics, 2 Ingrid Street, Clapham 5062, South Australia
(08) 371 3755

New Zealand: Human Kinetics, P.O. Box 105-231, Auckland 1
(09) 309-2259

To my wife, Tina, for her unyielding support and patience. To my children, Marissa and Chris, for their understanding. To my parents, Ray and Sandy, for their sacrifice and continued support. And to the good Lord who helps keep it all in perspective.

—SRT

To my parents, Robin and Susan, who started me down the right road and gave me educational freedom; to my mentor, Tab Blackburn, who has continued to give me professional direction; to my colleague and coauthor, Steve Tippett, who put up with countless rewrites and missed deadlines; and finally, to my wife, Cissy, whose love and understanding have helped to sustain my passion for education.

—MLV

CONTENTS

◆◆◆

Preface   vii

Part I   Using Functional Progressions for Rehabilitation   **1**

Chapter 1   Components of Functional Progression   **3**

Historical Perspective   3
Program Benefits   4
Program Prerequisites   6
Program Progression   8
Program Assessment   9
Integration With Formal Rehabilitation   9
Special Concerns   10
The Basic Program   10

Chapter 2   Neurophysiology of Functional Exercise   **19**

Motor Control and Learning   19
Sensory Input for Motor Control   19
Historical Perspective   22
Balance and Kinesthetic Awareness   25

Chapter 3   Functional Testing   **29**

Functional Testing Versus Functional Progression   29
Functional Testing Versus Functional Training   29
Why Perform Functional Testing?   30
When Should Functional Testing Be Performed?   31
Progression of Functional Testing   32
Bilateral and Unilateral Support Drills (Loaded)   38
Bilateral and Unilateral Nonsupport Drills   39
Agility Drills   42

Part II   Functional Progression for Specific Sports   **45**

Chapter 4   Collision and Contact Sports   **47**

Collision Sports   47
Contact Sports   47
Rehabilitation Concerns   47
Lower Extremity   48
Upper Extremity   53
Special Considerations   61

Chapter 5   Combat Sports   **63**

    Striking Functional Progressions   63
    Nonstriking Functional Progressions   67
    Special Concerns   71

Chapter 6   Jump Training   **73**

    Principles of Plyometric Training   74
    Program Development   77
    Plyometric Program Design   79
    Plyometric Training Guidelines   80

Chapter 7   Running Activities   **83**

    Functional Progression for Distance Runners   84
    Functional Progression for Sprinters   87

Chapter 8   Throwing Activities   **91**

    Repetitive Stress   91
    Rehabilitation   93
    Simulated Game Situations   94

Glossary   101

References   105

Index   111

About the Authors   119

PREFACE

◆◆◆

Fully preparing an injured athlete to return to formal competition means more than following a checklist of rigid, step-by-step procedures. Believing that an athlete is ready to return to play after merely satisfying clinical goals is a mistake that can result in reinjury or even the premature end of a career.

An athlete's full recovery and confidence in returning to play require a rehabilitation program that stresses a specific, gradual return to activity. *Functional Progressions for Sport Rehabilitation* gives you the tools to develop such a program.

Sport physical therapists, athletic trainers, and sports medicine specialists will find this book their most complete guide to the step-by-step progressions for rehabilitating injuries in major sports. We explain rehabilitation principles that can supplement your athletic injury program, and we detail the physiological and psychological principles underlying the steps in readying an injured athlete for competition.

In this book we discuss the basic components of a functional progression program and then delve into the prerequisites, the principles, and the physical and psychological benefits of functional progression.

Because most sport movement patterns occur in a closed kinetic chain, the International Knee Society suggests closed-chain functional testing after injury to the anterior cruciate ligament. We therefore present closed-chain exercise concepts and the neurophysiological basis of closed-chain activities as they relate to functional progression. Functional testing relates closely to functional progression drills yet remains its own area; we discuss thoroughly the similarities and differences between the two.

Finally, we categorize a myriad of sports and place each category into a model functional progression. Each model gives the framework to establish a functional progression program. We encourage you to tailor the programs to meet the needs of your own injured athletes.

We hope that through *Functional Progressions for Sport Rehabilitation*, you come to understand functional progression and functional testing and discover a handy reference for a variety of popular sporting activities. We want this book to be a catalyst that stimulates you to build on the model programs and, in turn, to provide your patients with the most comprehensive sport rehabilitation program possible.

PART I
Using Functional Progressions for Rehabilitation

◆◆◆

Your anterior cruciate ligament reconstruction patient has finally come to the last scheduled rehabilitation visit. It has been a long 7 months since surgery, and you feel a much deserved sense of accomplishment. Things have gone very well since the cruciate was replaced with the central third of the patellar tendon.

Your patient's active range of motion in the involved knee is symmetrical with the noninvolved knee, there are no complaints of patellofemoral pain, swelling is down, and the latest isokinetic values are excellent. You have achieved your clinical goals and are ready to discharge the patient from your care.

This is an all-too-familiar scenario. Once clinical goals of physical therapy are met, the patient is sent back to activities that may have caused the injury. Is this undesirable? Certainly not. Just as functional independence is a goal for all patients, returning the rehabilitated athlete to sporting activities is also a worthwhile effort. If you believe the athlete is ready to return to sports after merely satisfying clinical goals, however, you are sorely mistaken. As you will see in the following chapters, a series of events must lead the athlete from formal rehabilitation back to sports.

Chapter 1 will provide a brief historical review of the concept of functional progression, the principles governing functional rehabilitation, and guidelines to design a progression of functional activities, as well as an understanding of the physical and psychological benefits for you and the athletes under your care. Chapter 2 provides an in-depth review of proprioception and balance, with special attention to the afferent biology of a joint. Chapter 3 deals with functional testing, a vital concept to incorporate into rehabilitation programs. Use these three introductory chapters as a basis to tailor functional progression programs for specific sporting activities.

CHAPTER 1

◆◆◆

Components of Functional Progression

After a person who does industrial work has completed a clinical rehabilitation program, the therapist dealing with this patient would not dream of returning him or her to work without appropriate work hardening. In a work hardening program, the rehabilitation professional prepares the worker to return to the job by stressing the particular patient's work-related activities. The same should occur with the injured athlete. After attaining the clinical goals, the athlete is no more ready to return to competition than is the worker who has not undergone work hardening. Work hardening is an individualized final preparation that allows a worker to gear up for a return to the workplace. *Functional progression* is the series of sport-specific, basic movement patterns graduated according to the difficulty of the skill and the athlete's tolerance. The end goal of functional progression is an athlete's timely and safe return to competition.

Functional progression is a vital component of a conscientious return-to-sport program. Including functional progression in treatment is a sign of a prudent rehabilitation professional. Of utmost importance is that the athlete advances one step at a time. Function within a given sport must be broken down into basic skills and movements that are progressed gradually as the athlete tolerates. As the athlete reacquires the skills relevant to her or his sport, appropriate safeguards against further injury must be taken.

At the heart of functional progression is the *SAID* principle (Kegerreis, 1983). SAID is an acronym for Specific Adaptations to Imposed Demands. In a nutshell, this means that all rehabilitation, including functional progression, should be geared toward the demands that will be placed on the individual upon returning to his or her previous function. Accordingly, an athlete should not be rehabilitated in the same way as a nonathlete with

the same problem. Athletes stress particular body parts in a way that nonathletes do not. An effective rehabilitation program must prepare each individual for the demands that will be placed on the injured area once the program has been completed.

Inherent to a sound functional progression program is setting rehabilitation goals that recognize the demands of the specific sport. Demands placed on an American-football player, for instance, differ from those placed on a volleyball player. American football stresses speed and strength in a collision sport, whereas volleyball demands vertical power in a noncollision sport. So the functional progression program for players of these two sports will be dramatically different. Taking this a step further, the demands placed on an American-football quarterback vary from the demands placed on an American-football lineman. Most important to the quarterback position are speed and agility, whereas the emphasis for the lineman is on strength. Once again, the functional progression program for these two athletes must be different. A sound functional progression program needs to break down each athlete's role in his or her sport. Once the specific activity has been broken down into required fundamental movements, the athlete's injured body part is stressed progressively until function is adequate for the athlete to return to sport-specific demands.

◆ Historical Perspective

Although functional progression is not common to all sport rehabilitation programs, the concept is not a new one. Almost 20 years ago, Yamamoto, in a work coauthored by Feagin, described a functional progression program used in the rehabilitation of injured West Point cadets (Yamamoto, Hartman, Feagin, & Kimball, 1975). Emphasis in this program was placed on restoring agility through dynamic exercise after knee injury, versus what the authors termed a static exercise program. Kegerreis added specific movement patterns and skills to the program and introduced the importance of addressing the psychological needs of the injured athlete. He also addressed the scientific principles that play an important role in functional progression, specifically healing time constraints and proprioception. Specificity of the functional progression program was given high priority as well. The need to break down sport-specific functions to be gradually addressed within rehabilitation was put into perspective very well by Kegerreis, Malone, and McCarroll (1984) and by Kegerreis and Wetherald (1987).

♦ Program Benefits

Benefits of a sound functional progression program fit into two categories: those afforded the athlete, and those afforded the professional overseeing the sport rehabilitation program. Certainly, by benefitting the athlete, a sound functional progression program in turn indirectly benefits those responsible for the athlete's care. However, for the sake of discussion, benefits of functional progression that primarily affect the athlete will be separated from those that primarily affect the rehabilitation professional. Functional progression benefits, as they relate to the athlete and the rehabilitation team member, can be further broken down into physical benefits and psychological benefits.

Physical Benefits for the Sport Participant

During the healing process, injured tissue must be stressed according to the manner in which it functions. Stress imparted to the tissue must be sufficient to encourage healing but not so stressful as to inhibit healing. Following is discussion of the physiologic principles governing the healing process, as well as the physical benefits of the functional progression program.

Promotes Healing

Looking at functional progression through the eyes of the athlete, perhaps the most obvious benefit is the break-up of the monotony of traditional rehabilitation. Athletes appreciate performing activities related to function. Of course they are also pleased

to know that by performing these skills they are facilitating the healing of the injured body part.

Let's look at a basketball player rehabilitating an inversion ankle sprain. So far, the rehabilitation program has progressed through the acute phase; edema has been reduced, pain eliminated, and range of motion re-established. Weight-bearing status is full; resistance applied to the ankle evertors and dorsiflexors is tolerated and has been progressed from submaximal to maximal efforts. Now early in the functional progression program, the athlete is ready for simple jumping and hopping drills. These jumping activities are seen by the athlete as more closely related to function than the theraband strengthening exercises were, so the athlete is encouraged in the rehabilitation process. Of course the more stimulating activities are also facilitating the healing process.

At the heart of the physical benefits of functional progression are Davis's Law and Wolf's Law. These two physiologic principles state that soft tissue and bone respectively heal according to the manner in which they are stressed (Gould & Davies, 1985). Healing tissue responds to stress by reacting along the lines of the given stress. For optimum healing, tissue must be stressed gradually to accept a given force. If during rehabilitation healing tissue is not stressed in the way required of it before injury, the tissue will not be ready to fully accept preinjury requirements. Making the soft tissue accept this stress during rehabilitation will lead to strengthening of the tissue. Wolf's Law states that the same principle applies to healing bone. Take our previous example of the inversion sprain. If the athlete had been allowed to return to basketball after completing straight plane theraband resisted activities only, the healing lateral ankle ligaments would not have been stressed to provide for optimum healing required for basketball activities.

The first physical benefit of functional progression for the athlete is facilitation of the healing process. By applying the principles of Davis's Law and Wolf's Law, injured tissue is stressed to ready itself to accept forces required in sport, thus making the tissue stronger and more resilient. Without functional progression, injured tissue is not stressed to heal itself sufficiently for sport participation.

Maximizes Postinjury Performance

The second physical benefit afforded the athlete who participates in a comprehensive functional progression program is postinjury performance enhancement. During the successful completion of the functional progression program, the athlete proceeds from simple, safe skills to complex skills that more closely mimic competition. The differences in the performance of an athlete who has not undergone adequate functional progression training and an athlete who is prepared for a return to sport are readily apparent. Typically, performance of the person who has not taken part in the functional progression program is characterized by inadequate speed, strength, and/or endurance in a given sport skill. This is especially true as the degree of difficulty of a skill or the duration of participation is increased. The athlete who returns prematurely to competition usually favors the injured area and ends up either voluntarily or involuntarily being removed from competition. On the other hand, the athlete who has completed a functional progression program usually performs on the same level as the noninjured. Normal, unencumbered postinjury performance is the goal of the functional progression program.

Psychological Benefits for the Athlete

Any health care professional who has assisted in sport rehabilitation knows that the psyche deserves as much attention as the physical body. Helping the athlete return to competition with confidence after an injury is clearly a vital concern.

Minimizes the Stress of Being Injured

As if the physical problems the athlete must deal with after an injury aren't enough—he or she must confront the psychological effects as well. Sport psychologists have studied and documented the emotional reactions of athletes who have been injured (Bloomfield, Fricker, & Fitch, 1992; Nideffer, 1983). Often, removing an athlete from a sport after an injury can be devastating. For some people, sport is the most important thing in life. Taking sport away from such people can completely disrupt their lives. So, of course, the sooner they can resume normal activities, the better for their peace of mind.

Certainly not all cases are this drastic. For most people, sport is an important part of their life, not their entire existence. However, most people will experience similar psychological responses when removed from sport participation due to injury. Questions such as "What will I be like?" and "Will I be able to function?" are normal, and through the course of functional progression, these questions are answered.

Athletic endeavors, especially in the team setting, provide the athlete with a comfort zone. Injury removes the individual from this zone. It is in the athlete's best interest to return to the team setting as soon as possible. The comradeship of teammates or fellow sport enthusiasts is but one of the many positives of sport participation. When an injured individual can no longer interact with others in a sport environment, the individual may feel deprived. With such a patient, you must address the special psychological needs as well as the physical needs. One way of addressing psychological needs is to involve the athlete in functional progression.

As you will see, functional progression drills are introduced during rehabilitation as soon as the sport participant is ready. Those involved in team sports should be encouraged to perform these drills during regular practice sessions. When appropriate (e.g., with stretching exercises), the individual can perform the drills alongside noninjured teammates. When teammates are doing drills that the injured person is not ready for, functional progression drills can be performed at the same time somewhere else.

Returning the athlete to the familiar environment as soon as possible minimizes the stress of not fitting in due to injury. But it is important to remember that the athlete must be sufficiently rehabilitated before you consider returning her or him to competition.

Enhances Self-Confidence

Just as feelings of deprivation are normal for the injured person, feelings of uncertainty are also common. During rehabilitation, the injured person has to wonder how postrehabilitation function will compare to preinjury function. Extraneous pressures may be placed on the individual to recover well enough to maintain a starting position on the team, to keep a scholarship, or, in the case of a professional, to continue to earn a living.

As the athlete responds to rehabilitation, functional progression activities are introduced that prepare the individual for competition. It goes without saying that preparation enhances confidence. If the individual tolerates a graduated series of progressively difficult drills, self-confidence improves right along with specific sport function. The ideal functional progression program will ready the athlete for any situation he or she may encounter after returning to sport. The key here is that the person tackles each of the steps in a controlled, supervised functional progression program before being asked to perform competitively. Therefore, the athlete enters the competitive arena confident that function will be up to playing standards.

Benefits for the Rehabilitation Professional

Because you as the rehabilitation professional are not the injured party, the benefits you derive from effective rehabilitation are not physical, but psychological. Let's examine the benefits that you receive when you put your injured athlete through a functional progression program.

Gauges of Progress

Perhaps your most pertinent benefit of functional progression is your ability to gauge your athlete's tolerance to functional activity. (Whereas you can exercise the injured athlete on an isokinetic machine indefinitely and not even begin to address function.) More important, by having the injured person proceed through functional progression, you constantly have an accurate assessment of the individual's tolerance to a given activity. Tolerance to the functional progression program provides you a sport-specific gauge of progress. On page 8 you will find concrete guidelines governing advancement or curtailment of the functional progression program.

Establishes a Bridge to Participation

Hand in hand with providing a gauge of progress, functional progression also provides a sport-specific bridge for formal clinic-based rehabilitation to sport participation. This is essential in terms of Wolf's Law and Davis's Law, as healing tissue needs sport-specific activity to ready itself for actual sport performance. But functional progression offers a series of activities based on function that facilitates the athlete's transition from the acquisition of clinic-based goals to sport-specific goals. Depending on the individual's tolerance of the functional progression program, you can have a better idea of when she or he will be able to safely return to sports.

◆ Program Prerequisites

Functional progression drills are the activities that bridge the gap between clinic-based rehabilitation and sport function. But when is the individual ready to shift from traditional rehabilitation to functional progression activities? The answer: only *after* he or she has satisfied all clinic-based rehabilitation goals. Specifically, the injured area must

- not be swollen,
- not be painful,
- exhibit adequate range of motion,
- exhibit adequate strength, and
- not be stressed beyond what is allowed by healing time constraints.

Swelling

Along with pain, swelling is one of the most sensitive indicators of an overzealous rehabilitation program. Following an acute injury to a joint, there should be no swelling when functional progression is initiated. If swelling is present, partial weight-bearing activities that do not increase swelling should be stressed. Therapeutic modalities such as high volt galvanic stimulation, intermittent/constant compression, and/or cryotherapy should be emphasized.

Pain

Pain, nature's way of telling you that something is wrong, is the best way for determining if activity is too strenuous during rehabilitation. Functional progression drills are no exception; in a carefully advanced program, the athlete should experience no pain. If pain occurs with any rehabilitation activity, that particular activity should be avoided. Further injury is a distinct possibility. Also, pain is actually counterproductive to rehabilitation efforts because of reflex muscle inhibition. If pain is present, activity should be curtailed and analgesics, electrotherapeutic modalities (e.g., microamperage or transcutaneous electrical nerve stimulation), or cryotherapy should be employed.

Range of Motion

Full range of motion of the injured area must be present prior to initiating functional progression.

When dealing with the upper or lower extremity, consider full range of motion to be that which is present on the contralateral side. For spinal injuries, motion on each side of the joint axis should be symmetrical.

Remember—all joints have normal range of motion guidelines as well as normal end feels (e.g., soft tissue approximation, bone-to-bone, springy, etc.). However, it is also important to keep in mind that participants of certain sport activities may exhibit range of motion considered hypermobile or hypomobile in a nonsport participant or a player of another sport. In these cases, the demands placed on a joint may result in "abnormal" range of motion. A few common examples are the significantly increased shoulder external rotation of throwing athletes with a concomitant loss of internal rotation; the excessive lordosis and available extension of the low back in the female gymnast; and the extreme hip external rotation of the ballet dancer.

When range of motion deficits are present, functional progression activities should be deemphasized and active, active-assisted, or passive range of motion exercises stressed. As soon as range of motion is sufficient to allow unimpeded performance of the simplest functional progression activities, the formal program may be initiated.

Strength

Muscle strength that affords dynamic stability to any given joint must be adequate for the rigors of functional progression. An adequate strength base is absolutely essential for any sport activity. The same holds true for any functional progression program preparing an individual for sport competition. When an individual lacks sufficient muscle strength and power, functional progression drills are stress–failure overuse injuries waiting to happen.

When rehabilitating an injury of the lower extremity, strength should be returned to symmetry with the contralateral, uninjured leg. After injury to the upper extremity, equal strength on both sides may not be good enough. Ideally, strength of the athlete's dominant arm in throwing activities should be 10% to 15% greater than the nondominant arm. A stronger dominant than nondominant arm is especially important to the athlete who throws or plays racquet sports. Strength can be assessed in a number of ways. If you are using an isokinetic dynamometer, remember that results from one manufacturer's device will not apply to that of another. The same holds true if you attempt to extrapolate agonist:antagonist ratios, torque-output:body-weight ratios, and other generally accepted data (Cook, Gray, Savinar-Nogue, & Medeiros, 1987; Trundle, 1984; Walmsley & Szybbo, 1987; Wyatt & Edwards, 1981). Strength may also be assessed via hand-held dynamometers, but keep in mind the overall strength of the examiner, the joint position, and the location of applied resistance (McMahon, Burdett, & Whitney, 1992; Wadsworth & Krishan, 1987; Wikholw & Bohannon, 1991). Simple subjective manual muscle tests, functional testing (see chapter 3), and other standard methods may also be used to assist in determining strength.

Remember the specific strengthening goals that take priority when you are rehabilitating a specific injury. Muscle groups that should be emphasized in the sport rehabilitation program will be included when we discuss common injuries unique to a given sport (see chapters 4 through 8).

Healing Time Constraints

It is beyond this book's scope to discuss sequelae of all sport injuries as they relate to healing parameters. However, it is vital during every phase of rehabilitation not to stress healing tissue beyond its tolerance. Many factors play a direct role in how the sport participant responds after sport injury. These include the effects of immobilization after sport injury; the natural course after surgical and nonsurgical intervention; the condition of the injured tissue; the overall general conditioning of the individual prior to injury; and the age of the athlete (Barrack, Bruckner, Kneisl, Inman, & Alexander, 1990; Buckley, Barrack, & Alexander, 1989; Elmqvist, Lorentzon, Langstrom, & Fugl-Meyer, 1988; Harter, Osternig, Singer, James, Larson, & Jones, 1988; Indelicato, Hermansdorfer, & Huegel, 1990; Jokl, Kaplan, Stovell, & Keggi, 1987; Noyes, Torvik, Hyde, & DeLucas, 1974; Odensten, Lysholm, & Gillquist, 1985; Weiss, Lundberg, Hamberg, DeHaven, & Gillquist, 1989). You must consider all these variables and implement, monitor, and modify your functional progression program accordingly.

Here are some red flags to alert you that healing time constraints are being exceeded:

- The presence of or an increase in swelling
- The presence of or an increase in pain
- A loss of or a plateau in range of motion
- A loss of or a plateau in strength
- Documented increased laxity of a healing ligament

♦ Program Progression

Now that you have an idea of the basic prerequisites that individuals must meet prior to beginning a functional progression program, let's move ahead to the actual implementation. Of course we must always remember that each athlete is unique and requires a customized program.

Think of functional progression as progressing through elementary school. In grade school, basic skills are introduced and built on throughout the year. At regular intervals, tests are given, grades are assigned, and, at the end of the school year, the student either advances to the next grade or is retained to repeat the year over. Functional progression applies the same basic principles. Early in the program, simple skills are used as building blocks for the more advanced skills to come. Throughout the program the sport participant is evaluated and reevaluated. If no problems are encountered, progression to the next step is allowed. However, if problems arise at a given stage, the person remains there until the problem is solved. He or she can proceed to the next stage only after preceding skills are performed satisfactorily and are well tolerated.

Here are the guidelines governing the advancement of the functional progression program:

- Initiate skills at a slow speed and progress to faster speeds.
- Initiate skills that are simple and progress to more difficult skills.
- Initiate skills at short distances and progress to longer distances.
- Initiate skills unloaded (unresisted) and progress to loaded (resisted) skills.

Slow Speeds Progressed to Fast Speeds

Put simply: You have to crawl before you can walk. Initially, speed should be kept slow with emphasis on proper form and skill execution. As the skill is mastered, it becomes more automatic, requiring less volitional and conscious effort. Once the skill can be performed properly, the speed may be increased. For example, jogging must be with symmetrical weight bearing and weight shift prior to running, which in turn is required prior to sprinting. The same principle applies to throwing, rowing, swimming, cycling, and other activities.

Simple Skills Progressed to Difficult Skills

Inherent to this guideline is a working knowledge of the skills required for a given sport activity. A coach who knows the athlete's sport can be especially helpful in applying this guideline. If you do not know the specific requirements of the given sport, admit your limitations, and try to become better informed. Other options are to send the athlete to a professional with better knowledge in the area or to work closely with the athlete's coach in a joint effort. Examples in which this guideline comes into play are simple countering moves in wrestling, the intricacies involved in diving or gymnastics, or the footwork required in the football offensive backfield.

Short Distances Progressed to Longer Distances

Not only does skill enter into this area, but now sport-specific anaerobic and aerobic endurance must be considered. Function must not be only automatic and efficient but must also be able to be performed for the duration of time required by a given sport. Without an adequate anaerobic or aerobic base, function not only suffers but the athlete is at greater risk of reinjury as the duration of activity increases.

Unloaded Activities Progressed to Loaded Activities

Unloaded skills are those in which no outside resistance is applied to the athlete. These are contrasted with *loaded* activities in which extra resistance is added to the individual. Examples of unloaded activities are running, assuming the down position in wrestling, and an American-football player practicing agility drills while running with the football. Loaded activities are the same runner running with a weighted vest, the wrestler in a down position with another wrestler on top of him, and the football player being tackled by defenders. When progressing to loaded activities, extra care should be taken by the rehabilitation professional, the coach, or a trained observer to regulate and supervise the athlete.

◆ Program Assessment

Now that you know the guidelines governing the progression of the program, we need to look at those red flags that indicate the individual is not ready to advance in the functional progression. As trained health care professionals, we are keenly trained in observation skills. These skills are of utmost importance in monitoring the functional progression program. And when you are not able to personally monitor the athlete performing functional progression skills, it is crucial that you alert the athlete to the signs indicating that a component of the program has not been tolerated and that the athlete should not proceed.

In assessing the athlete throughout the functional progression program, refer to the three Cs:

- Carriage
- Confidence
- Control

The individual must assume the posturing and positioning required to carry the body smoothly through each step of the program. Weight shift, weight acceptance, and symmetry of movement are all indicators of *carriage*. As the individual attempts each step, *confidence* is displayed by facial expression and by the speed and deliberateness with which a skill is performed. An uncertain sport participant is asking for reinjury. *Control* is exemplified by smooth, unrestricted, automatic movement with precise performance of a given task.

Besides the three Cs, other indicators that the individual cannot tolerate a particular component of the functional progression include the following:

- Perceived instability of the involved area during performance of a skill
- Pain present during the activity
- Athlete anxiety when a new skill is introduced
- Athlete's inability to perform the skill immediately preceding in the progression
- Pain, swelling, or decreased range of motion following the task

◆ Integration With Formal Rehabilitation

Before we look at the basic functional progression program, you must first understand how the program is to be integrated with the formal rehabilitation program. As you discovered on page 6, the functional progression program should begin after range of motion and strength are adequate and pain and edema have subsided. This does not mean that the entire formal rehabilitation program must be completed prior to initiating functional progression. As the athlete accomplishes goals established in the formal rehabilitation program, functional progression drills compatible with the person's physical status may be implemented. Take our earlier example of the athlete with an inversion ankle sprain. Pain and swelling are under control; range of motion and strength are coming along nicely but are still subpar. Gait is without an assistive device and is done without a limp. You need not wait until strength is normal and range of motion is symmetrical with the opposite side to start simple weight-bearing drills in the functional progression (e.g., step-ups), if the individual is able to perform them without pain.

The best rule to apply when implementing any functional progression drill is to break the drill down to its basic components and ascertain that the individual can perform these skills. To begin skills that stress bilateral support (weight-bearing on both legs), the individual must be able to walk without a limp, exhibit normal and symmetrical weight shift, and demonstrate normal stride length and cadence. If any of these abilities are absent, it is too early to initiate bilateral support drills.

When stressing functional progression drills involving unilateral support, make sure that the individual can bear full weight solely on the involved side and can raise fully up onto the toes. Again, if this simple component of unilateral support is absent, functional progression drills involving weight bearing on one leg only should not be performed.

Your observation of the athlete must be sharp to assess progression readiness and to critically analyze performance. If there is no pain and if the athlete exhibits carriage, control, and confidence, the skill can be initiated. On the other hand, if there is a breakdown in any of the three Cs, if there is pain, or if there are detrimental effects after the drill, the skill should not be performed.

The athlete progressing toward a return to competition may reach a point when he or she can participate in most practice drills but still need to perform a component of the functional progression program as well. For example, a basketball player may have progressed through jumping and hopping drills but not yet be ready for weaving and cutting drills. In this case the player may participate in all team rebounding and tipping drills but should not scrimmage. In such a situation, all functional progression activities should be performed after the team participation drills. This will minimize the risk of reinjury due to fatigue during participation drills following the more aggressive functional progression drills.

♦ Special Concerns

Of special concern is the use of any therapeutic modalities or special added support of the injured area during functional progression activities. If special stretching is required of the involved body part, moist heat (or deep heat if indicated and available) may facilitate stretching. Certainly, any cryotherapy and/or compression if indicated after activity should also be employed.

Additional support may also be required for the injured area during functional progression. Such support ranges from neoprene sleeves to retain warmth to ankle taping or bracing to a sophisticated functional knee brace. As always, the individual's unique circumstances should dictate which supportive measures are used, if any.

♦ The Basic Program

Now that you are aware of the fundamental premises governing functional progression, the program's prerequisites, and the reasons for instituting a functional progression program, an example of the program can be introduced. The following example is of the most basic functional progression program upon which sport-specific skills need to be added. As you will see in Part 2, you will need to augment this fundamental program to satisfy the needs of the specific athlete.

Also, understand that the entire program is not meant for all of your injured athletes. Often, an athlete will be beyond a given skill when you enter the rehabilitation scene. Whether a particular step is applicable depends on the individual. For example, a specific step of the functional progression program may not be applicable

- because the athlete's sport does not require performance of a given skill, or
- because the athlete's condition supersedes the physical demands of the skill.

So, familiarize yourself with the following program and use it as a guideline. If you feel that a particular step does not apply to the individual you are treating, omit the step or modify it. Later chapters on specific sports will provide the detailed, sport-specific drills you require. The basic functional progression program that follows is geared toward lower extremity problems. Most sports involve the lower extremity functions of running, jumping, hopping, cutting, etc. For sports that single out such upper extremity functions as swinging, throwing, and striking, refer to the chapters dealing with specific activities.

Bilateral Support Drills (Mini-Squats)

Once the athlete can bear full weight on the involved lower extremity, mini-squats may be initiated. A mini-squat is performed with the feet shoulder-width apart and the body weight centered over a stable base of support. Bearing weight symmetrically, and with the trunk upright over the legs, the individual flexes at the hips and knees into a partial squat. The squat can be carried down to a position in which the thighs are parallel with the floor, or it can be stopped at a prior point (see Figure 1.1).

If care must be taken to avoid anterior translation of the tibia (e.g., anterior cruciate defi-

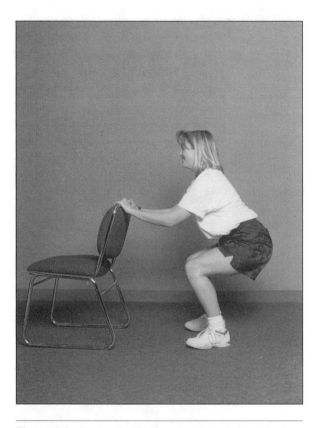

Figure 1.1 Knees should always remain behind the toes when attempting to protect the anterior cruciate ligament. Ideally, tibia should remain perpendicular to the floor. Manual support may be utilized for balance if required.

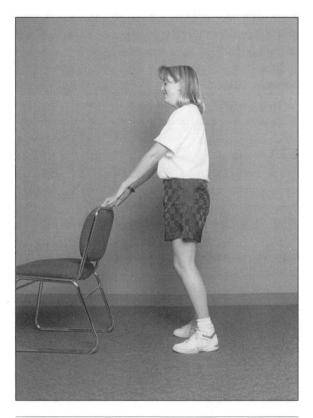

Figure 1.2 Manual support is allowed for balance only. Watch for pelvic symmetry as body weight is smoothly lowered onto the heel of the noninvolved leg and as the individual returns to a position about 5 degrees from full extension.

ciency), position of the tibia may be of prime concern. A perpendicular position of the tibia takes advantage of the normally occurring 7 degree posterior tilt of the tibial plateau (Turek, 1984). Maintaining the tibia perpendicular to the floor also helps to minimize patellofemoral reaction forces. Telling the individual always to keep the knees posterior to the toes while performing the mini-squat will help assure normal positioning. If anterior translation or retropatellar compression is not of concern, the individual may be allowed greater closed chain ankle dorsiflexion and knee flexion. During the mini-squat, emphasis is placed on a controlled eccentric quadriceps contraction. The athlete lowers for a 2 count and after another 2 count returns to a position approximately 5 degrees from full extension (see Figure 1.2).

The mini-squat enhances weight bearing, which facilitates feedback from the mechanoreceptors located in proximal and distal joint structures. The athlete can perform 2 to 3 sets of 15 repetitions and progress to 30 repetitions as tolerated, but perhaps a better option is to exercise for a set period of time. Early in the program, a range of 15 to 30 seconds is an adequate amount of time. As individual tolerance dictates, time can be increased to 2 minutes. Whether during functional testing or functional progression, it is important to carefully watch closed kinetic chain activities. It is only through careful observation that improper substitutions for the desired movement can be detected. Once undesired movements are noted, the exercise should be terminated. This holds true whether the skill is performed for repetitions or for time.

Unilateral Support Drills (Step-Ups)

Think of a step-up as a unilateral mini-squat. In fact, the best way to begin the step-up portion of the functional progression is with a unilateral mini-squat. A mini-squat can be performed on the injured lower extremity emphasizing controlled hip and knee flexion, followed by a smooth return to the starting position just shy of full extension, as noted in Figure 1.3.

Once this skill is mastered, you may progress the athlete to a step-up. Step-ups can be performed in the sagittal plane (for a forward step-up) or in the transverse planes (for the more popular lateral step-up). Any stable object of appropriate height can be used as a step. Traditional stairs will do in a pinch but are sometimes too steep for the beginning step-up drills. A common footstool can also be used, but again, the height of the stool may be excessive for beginning step-ups. If necessary, use a stack of books, mats, aerobic steps, or a graduated series of wooden platforms (see Figure 1.4).

To eliminate pushing off with the noninvolved leg, start the step-up with the heel of the noninvolved foot on the floor. Using a 2 count, the individual shifts weight to the involved side and uses the involved lower extremity to raise the body onto the step. The knee is extended to approximately 5 to 10 degrees from neutral, held for a 2 count, and then flexed as weight is shifted toward the noninvolved side and the body weight is lowered back to the heel, as shown in Figure 1.5. An appropriate height to aim for is from 6 to 8 inches, but sometimes it is necessary to start lower. Taller individuals may require higher distances.

Another way to perform the step-up is to emphasize a quick weight shift from the involved to the

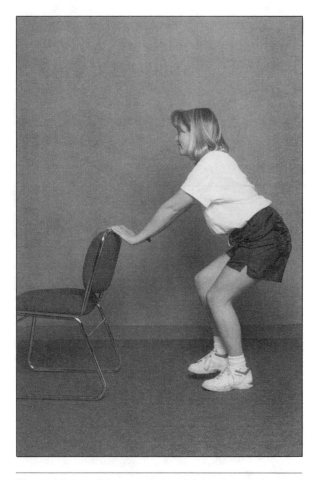

Figure 1.3   A mini-squat can be performed on the involved lower extremity only. Same form and movement pattern is emphasized as in the bilateral support mini-squat drill, but here on the involved leg only.

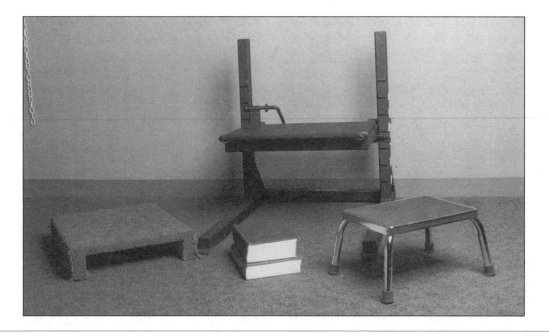

Figure 1.4   Many objects readily available around the clinic or training room may be used for step-ups. Care must be taken to assure that equipment is safe, and heights are progressed in a common-sense fashion.

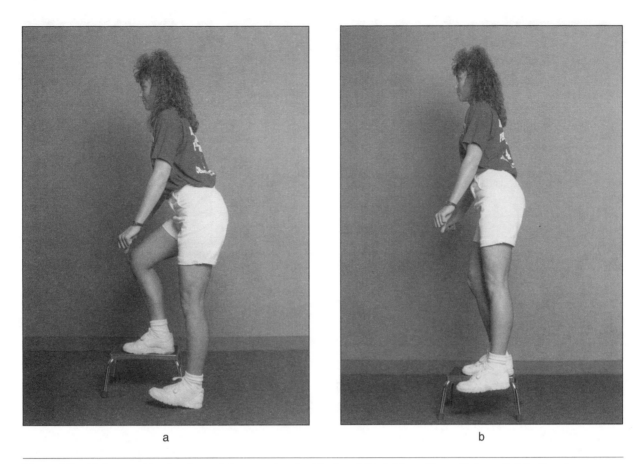

a

b

Figure 1.5   (a) Start position bearing weight on noninvolved heel, and (b) finish position with knee slightly flexed.

noninvolved leg. In this quick step-up, the involved lower extremity is made to both ascend and descend from the step. For this activity the starting position is the same as previously described. However, instead of the involved leg remaining alone on the step to support body weight, the noninvolved leg is also brought up to the step. The individual is then asked to step off of the opposite side of the step to the floor and bear the entire body weight on the involved lower extremity, as shown in Figure 1.6. This activity can also be performed with a forward step-up.

Bilateral Nonsupport Drills (Jumping)

Nonsupport drills refer to one or both feet being off the ground before returning to the ground. Bilateral nonsupport drills are those that involve jumping (Tippett, 1990a). They begin with both the involved and noninvolved lower extremity on the ground, followed by both legs leaving the ground, and then both legs landing on the ground again. Support drills use the effects of gravity as the stationary body imparts stress to the involved lower extremity.

In nonsupport drills the involved lower extremity must accept both the body's weight plus the added momentum as the athlete returns to the ground.

Jumping drills are best initiated by having the athlete jump forward and backward over a line drawn or taped on the floor. Emphasis is placed on landing on each side of the line as rapidly as possible, as shown in Figure 1.7a. Once front-to-back jumping is readily tolerated, side-to-side jumping is initiated (see Figure 1.7b).

After mastering straight plane forward/backward and lateral jumping, the athlete can begin diagonal patterns. To stress diagonal jumping drills, draw or tape on the floor two lines in the shape of a cross. These intersecting lines create four quadrants that can be numbered. The athlete is then given various sequences to perform (see Figure 1.8). For example, the first set may be 1,3,2,4 and the second set 1,4,2,3. Initially, emphasize jumping that minimizes height; as performance improves, the height of the jump can be increased.

Increase height by use of a rope, cones, lightweight bars, or other suitable materials (see Figure

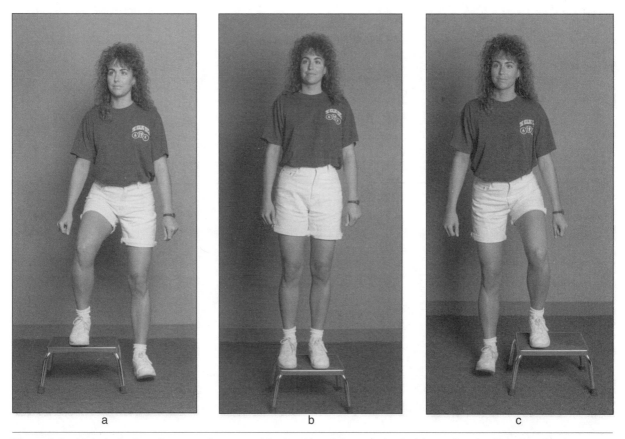

Figure 1.6   (a) As in the lateral step-up, the start position is with weight on the heel of the noninvolved leg. (b) After the step-up is performed, the noninvolved leg is brought up to the step. (c) The athlete then steps off of the opposite side of the step accepting full body weight on the involved lower extremity. The sequence is quickly repeated in the opposite direction.

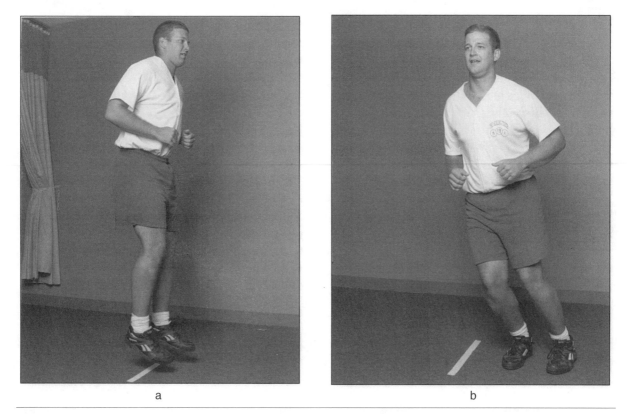

Figure 1.7   (a) Front-to-back line jumps and (b) side-to-side line jumps.

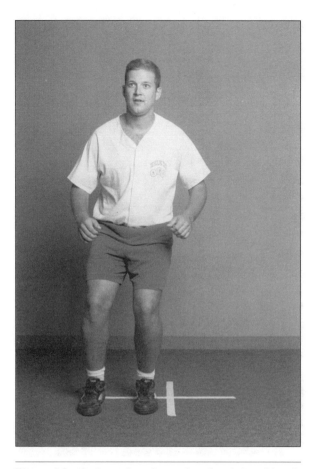

Figure 1.8 Each quadrant is numbered and the athlete is asked to perform bilateral or unilateral support drills, by jumping or hopping in a given sequence.

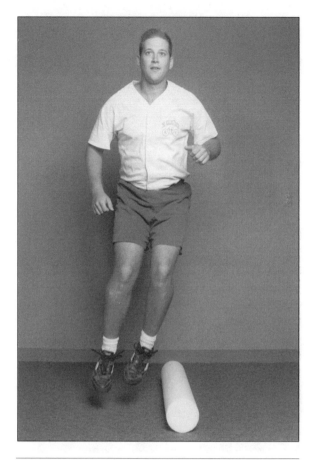

Figure 1.9 To add a vertical component to bilateral or unilateral support drills, the individual can jump or hop over a bar, cone, or other suitable object.

1.9). You can also increase difficulty by having the athlete cover a set distance by performing repetitive jumps. In this case, the athlete performs multiple response drills, which require added effort due to increased momentum. Such drills have a plyometric component and are valuable in the rehabilitation of the jumping athlete (see chapter 6).

Unilateral Nonsupport Drills (Hopping)

Just as support drills progress from bilateral to unilateral efforts, so do nonsupport drills. In hopping, the individual begins and ends the drill on one leg. All hopping drills are performed on the involved leg only and are progressed in the same manner as jumping (see Figure 1.10).

Acceleration/Deceleration Pivoting Drills

For those whose only activity performed is straight ahead running, a specific program to prepare for given distances and speeds can be instituted at this point. For guidelines for returning an athlete to running activities, see chapter 7. But for sports involving running along with stopping, cutting, pivoting, or jumping, additional drills must be added to the basic functional progression program.

Up to this point, emphasis has been on cardinal plane maneuvers performed in one place. Mini-squats, step-ups, jumping, and hopping are all done with the athlete repeating a single movement. The athlete has remained in the cardinal plane, performing mini-squats in the sagittal plane and step-ups in the sagittal and transverse planes. The only exception to this has been jumping and hopping drills performed in a diagonal. Because many sports involve running up and down a playing field with quick stops and starts and cuts and pivots as the athlete covers distance, the functional progression program must address these demands as well.

Figure-Eight Drills

A basic premise of the functional progression program is to advance the sport participant in a

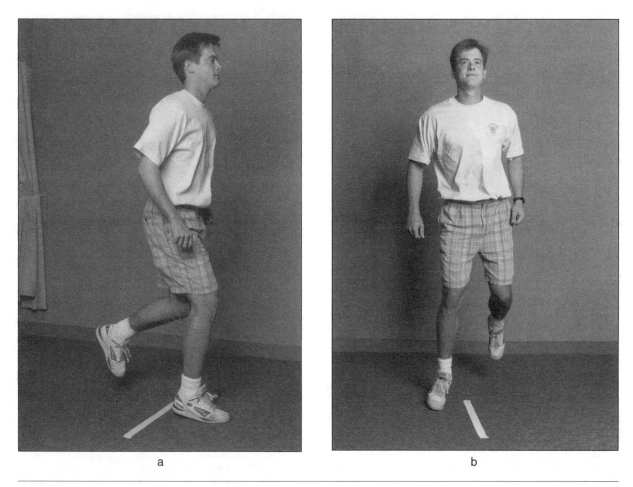

      a   b

Figure 1.10 (a) Front-to-back line hops and (b) side-to-side line hops.

graduated fashion. If a particular sport activity requires quick stops and sudden change of direction (cutting), the last thing you want to do is stress this activity immediately. Figure-eight drills are a good way to ease the individual into the demands of cutting. With figure-eights, the change of direction is more gradual, allowing the athlete to slowly build up to more strenuous cutting activities. To progress figure-eight drills, the distance the athlete must cover begins long and is progressed to shorter distances. This seems to contradict one of the guidelines of functional progression—namely, beginning with short distances and progressing to longer ones. But when you think about it, it makes perfect sense. By first covering a longer distance, a larger surface area is available for the athlete to perform the figure-eight. As the distance is decreased, a smaller area is available to weave through the figure. The shorter the distance, the tighter the figure-eight. Common progressions should be sport-specific—that is, distances covered should be simi-

lar to those required for the athlete's sport. If you are working with a basketball player, there is no need to cover a distance that a soccer player would need to cover.

 Common distances stressed usually begin with 40 yards. The athlete performs 10 repetitions of figure-eight running at half-speed (jogging). When the 10 repetitions are completed, a minute to 2-minute rest is allowed. After resting, the athlete increases to three-quarter speed (running), performs 10 repetitions, rests, and then completes the distance sprinting full speed. Again, after adequate recovery time, the distance is cut in half to 20 yards and the above sequence is repeated. Finally, the distance is decreased to 10 yards and the sequence is repeated again (see Figure 1.11). If the athlete will be required to perform backward running while weaving and cutting, the figure-eight sequence should also be performed backward. After progressing the athlete through the figure-eights, you can add more aggressive cutting maneuvers.

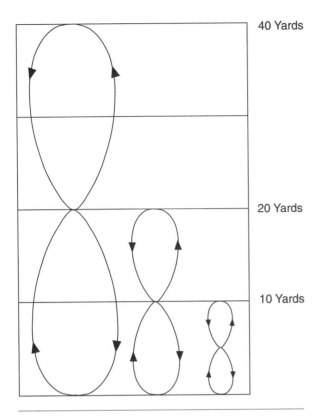

40 Yards

20 Yards

10 Yards

Figure 1.11   The distance should be adjusted for sport specificity (e.g., tennis or racquetball court, baseball or softball diamond).

Cutting Maneuver Drills

Let's look at things simply. An athlete changing direction requires only a few basic mechanisms. The athlete must either plant the right foot and cut right or left or plant the left foot and cut right or left. These two cutting maneuvers have been termed a *straight* cut (also called a *sidestep* cut by Cross, Gibbs, and Bryant, 1989) and a *crossover* cut (Kegerreis et al., 1984). A straight cut involves planting one leg, then pushing off this leg and cutting in the opposite direction (see Figure 1.12a). A crossover cut involves planting one leg and pivoting on it as the other leg crosses in front as the athlete cuts in the direction of the planted foot (see Figure 1.12b).

Remember—the functional progression program must be advanced gradually, and cutting maneuvers are no exception (Tippett, 1990b). Early cutting drills are performed with the participant approaching a predetermined spot at which the cut is to be performed. (A cone, line on the floor, or other marker can be used.) The athlete first jogs to the spot and performs the cut. This is followed by the athlete

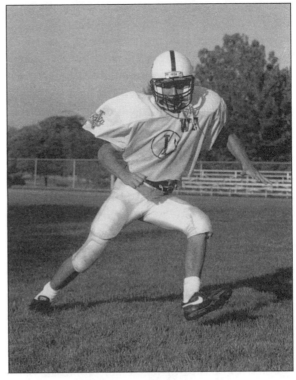

a

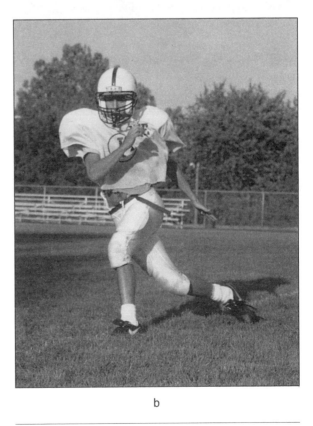

b

Figure 1.12   (a) Straight cut. The individual plants the foot of the involved leg and cuts to the same side of the planted foot. (b) Crossover cut. The individual plants the foot of the involved leg and cuts to the opposite side.

cutting at a half-speed sprint and then, finally, at a full-speed sprint. As with the figure-eight sequence, 10 repetitions with an appropriate rest are performed at each of the previously mentioned speeds.

Depending on the injury, straight cuts may precede crossover cuts, or vice versa. When we discuss specific sport injuries, this will make more sense. However, one quick example may help. A soccer player has suffered a sprain of the lateral collateral ligament of the knee. Because a crossover cut (varus stress) stresses the lateral ligaments greater than the medial ligaments, straight cuts should precede crossover cuts. Another way to gradually stress the healing tissue is to gradually increase the angle of the cut. If the individual cannot tolerate cutting at a 90-degree angle, begin at 45 degrees, progress to 60 degrees, and then finally try 90 degrees.

◆ Summary

In this important introductory chapter, we have explored the basics of functional progression. A brief history of functional progression has been provided to give perspective. The physical benefits to the athlete of postinjury performance and promoting healing were discussed, along with the psychological benefits for both you and the patient you treat. To assist you in implementing the program, vital prerequisites the athlete must meet before starting functional progression were also presented.

Table 1.1 is a skeleton outline to assist you in creating your own functional progression program. Having your athletes perform this basic program is a good way to begin work toward a return to competition. However, sport-specific function needs to be interjected into the program at the right time to ensure complete competition readiness. Sport-specific guidelines will be described in chapters 4 through 9. Prior to that, we need to take a deeper look at the neurophysiological basis on which functional activities are based. Once you have grasped the basics of functional progression and understand the scientific basis for the program, your imagination will be the only limit in designing and implementing functional progression programs for the athletes under your care.

Table 1.1 Sample Functional Progression

Unloaded activities	Loaded activities
Bilateral support drills	Single-plane one-on-one force delivery and force acceptance drills
Unilateral support drills	Multiplane one-on-one force delivery and force acceptance drills
Bilateral nonsupport drills	Single-plane two-on-one force delivery and force acceptance drills
Unilateral nonsupport drills	Multiplane two-on-one force delivery and force acceptance drills
Acceleration/deceleration pivoting drills	

CHAPTER 2

◆◆◆

Neurophysiology of Functional Exercise

Chapter 1 built a case for functional progression as the definitive rehabilitation step for returning a patient to sport activities. We saw that limiting rehabilitation to the traditional programs centered on the restoration of range of motion, muscle strength, and muscle endurance often results in an incomplete restoration of athletic ability. A common error is assuming that clinical programs using open kinetic-chain exercises with the distal segment free safely returns function. Research has proved that the body adapts to specific training demands. Athletes and patients cannot succeed if they have not been prepared to meet all the demands of the specific activity. This chapter will describe the neurophysiological rationale for including functional exercise in the total rehabilitation program.

◆ Motor Control and Learning

The ability to move is critical in all aspects of our lives, and our movements are more than mere coincidence in our daily routines. Researchers suggest that high cognitive skills in humans have evolved in order to master those movements essential to survival (Schmidt, 1988). How the central nervous system (CNS) interprets sensory information from the environment and the body and then controls the individual muscles and joints to produce coordinated movement is the science of *motor control*. The motor control system is designed to follow a stored sensory pattern. The mind compares the intent and production of a desired movement with stored information within the CNS, adjusting until any discrepancy in the movement meets the limits of performance allowed by the performer. As the individual reaches higher levels of motor control, these limits are systematically extended, allowing for finer coordinated control. Motor learning is the mind's attempt to teach the body conscious control

of a new movement or motor program. The axiom that "practice makes perfect" holds for motor learning or motor performance.

A specific motor learning task is maximally efficient when it runs its course automatically (Hellenbrandt, 1978). Successful repetition of a pattern of motion makes its performance progressively less difficult, requiring less concentration, until the pattern becomes automatic. When the pattern can be carried out with great ease, motor learning has occurred. Now the movement is controlled on the subcortical level, leaving the brain free to program new patterns of movement. These new movement patterns depend on the CNS's formation of new functional pathways. Repetitive activity results in a progressive decrease in the resistance at synapses in these patterns. Training for the new pattern of movement requires that the essential motion be carried out the same way many times. Skill progression is moving step-by-step from simple to more complex motions. For a rehabilitative program tailored to the specific demands on an individual, you should order the steps in a hierarchy and then have the patient perform them in a sequence that allows for acquiring or reacquiring the skill.

Cortical interference is the single greatest obstacle to motor learning (Hellenbrandt, 1978). For individuals to function in the real world, they must be able to interpret sensory motor information at the subcortical level. The development of a functional exercise program must center on finding the cues that will produce a functional decortication and get the patient's conscious mind out of the way.

◆ Sensory Input for Motor Control

Proprioception refers to all the neural inputs originating from the mechanoreceptors about the joint.

Sherrington first described the term *proprioception* in 1906 when he noted the presence of receptors in the joint capsular structures that were primarily reflexive. The typical mechanoreceptor ending is surrounded by specialized epithelial cells responsible for many of the responses from stimuli. These mechanoreceptors are biological transducers converting the mechanical distortion of the tissues into electrical activity and transmitting a neural signal back to the CNS.

Mechanoreceptors are specifically sensitive to changes originating in a joint's tissues, rather than external stimuli: hence, the classification as proprioceptors. Receptors about the joint are stimulated or distorted by the biomechanical forces that accompany soft tissue—stretching, compression, and fluid pressure changes. Receptor discharge varies according to the distortion's intensity. This neural signal is a repetitive discharge of action potentials whose rate directly relates to the intensity of the stimulus.

Once stimulated, mechanoreceptors are able to adapt. With constant stimulation the frequency of neural impulses decreases. The functional implication here is that mechanoreceptors detect change and rates of change, as opposed to steady-state conditions (Schulte & Happel, 1990). The receptors can be either rapidly or slowly adapting, which also has implications in their functional role. This input is then analyzed in the CNS for joint position and movement (Willis & Grossman, 1981). The status of the articular structures is sent to the CNS so that information regarding static versus dynamic conditions, equilibrium versus disequilibrium, or biomechanical stress and strain relations may be evaluated. Once processed and evaluated, this proprioceptive information becomes capable of influencing muscle tone, motor execution programs, and cognitive somatic perceptions or kinesthetic awareness (Rowinski, 1990). Proprioceptive information also protects the joint from damage caused by movement exceeding the normal physiologic range of motion and helps to determine the appropriate balance of synergistic and antagonistic forces.

All of this information helps to generate a somatosensory image within the CNS. It then becomes apparent that the soft tissues surrounding a joint serve a double purpose: They provide biomechanical support to the bony partners making up the joint, keeping them in relative anatomical alignment, and through the extensive afferent neurological network, they provide valuable proprioceptive information.

Classification of Mechanoreceptors

Mechanoreceptors were first identified in the structures surrounding a joint in the mid-1800s, shortly after the development of the compound microscope. Since that time, many studies have documented the presence of mechanoreceptors in virtually all joints.

Joint receptors have been classified according to function and morphological appearance (Rowinski, 1990). Receptors can be further subdivided and categorized by location (Schulte & Happel, 1990):

- Articular
- Deep (muscle-tendon related)
- Superficial (cutaneous)

Articular Mechanoreceptors

The articular mechanoreceptors are located within the joint capsule, ligaments, and any intra-articular structures (i.e., menisci) within the joint (Zimny, 1988). Studies of the human (Zimny, 1988) and animal (O'Conner, 1984) knee menisci have demonstrated that the same types of mechanoreceptors found in the ligaments are also found in the outer and middle third of the meniscal cartilage.

Ruffini Endings

Ruffini endings are found in the superficial fibrous layers of the joint capsule, and with greatest density in the capsular regions of the proximal joints in the area of greatest capsular stress. Occasionally, they are found on the surfaces of extrinsic ligaments but not on collateral ligaments (Freeman & Wyke, 1967b). These mechanoreceptors have a low mechanical threshold for stimulation and are very slow to adapt to a stimulus. Ruffini endings are relatively silent during the midrange of joint motion and are thought to be incapable of signaling joint position (Willis & Grossman, 1981). In addition, Ruffini endings are sensitive to changes in intracapsular fluid pressure.

Pacinian Corpuscles

Pacinian corpuscles are mechanoreceptors that also have a low mechanical threshold for stimulation but which rapidly adapt to a stimulus. They are found in the deeper layers of the joint capsule near the junction of the capsule and the synovial border in the stratum synovium. They lie in close approximation with the blood vessels supplying the synovial membrane. In contrast to the Ruffini endings, Pacinian corpuscles have their greatest density in the distal joints. The Pacinian corpuscles are silent in the immobile joint but activate at the onset or cessation of movement. They respond to high velocity changes in joint position with either acceleration or deceleration. Synovial mechanical distortion can also lead to activation of the Pacinian corpuscles. They may be sensitive to rapid contractile events of the adjacent muscles, as well.

Golgi-Like Receptors

There are two types of Golgi mechanoreceptors: Golgi-Mazzoni corpuscles and Golgi ligament endings. Golgi-Mazzoni corpuscles are located along the inner surface of the joint capsule between the fibrous layer and the subcapsular fibroadipose tissue. They have a low mechanical threshold and are slow in adapting to a stimulus. They respond to perpendicular compression of the joint capsule and are insensitive to capsular stretching.

Golgi ligament endings are found in both the extrinsic and intrinsic ligaments. Their greatest density is clustered adjacent to the bony attachments of the ligaments. They too have a low mechanical threshold and are slow in adapting to tension or stretch on the ligaments. The Golgi ligament endings are relatively silent when the joint is immobile. When the joint ligaments become stretched, which can occur at the extreme ends of joint motion, these Golgi receptors become active.

Nociceptors

Free nociceptive nerve endings also provide neurosensory information. Though these receptors differ in that they do not possess a well-differentiated corpuscular end organ, they are found in all areas of the joint except in the menisci. They are slow to adapt to biomechanical stress and have a low- to high-mechanical threshold.

Deep Muscle-Tendon Related Receptors

The deep muscle-tendon related receptors include muscle spindles, Golgi tendon organs, and pressure pain endings.

Muscle Spindle

The muscle spindle is a complex receptor located within the muscle fibers, with greatest density near the belly of the muscle. The muscle spindle is considered the third most complex sensory organ, after the eye and the ear (Schulte & Happel, 1990). The spindle's main function is to monitor the length of the muscle in which it is embedded and thus function as a stretch receptor. Once stimulated, muscle spindles initiate a contraction that will reduce the stretch imposed on the muscle. An example of the muscle spindle response is the stretch or the knee-jerk reflex.

Muscle spindles lie parallel to the normal or extrafusal muscle fibers. The fibers that contain the muscle spindles themselves are called intrafusal fibers. Within the intrafusal fibers lies a central sensory region sensitive to stretching or a change in length. When a muscle stretches, the muscle spindle, by virtue of lying parallel, also stretches. The sensory portion of the spindle sends an impulse to the spinal cord and synapses with an alpha motoneuron. The alpha motoneuron then causes a response contraction of the muscle. In addition, other impulses are sent to the antagonistic muscles that cause an inhibition. The resultant reaction is *contraction*, or shortening of the elongated muscle, thereby relieving the stretch.

Golgi Tendon Organs

Golgi tendon organs are located in the tendon near the musculotendinous junction. They respond to both contraction and stretching of the muscular unit. Their main function is to monitor and respond to tension developed in the tendon. If this tension becomes excessive and potentially harmful, stimulation of the Golgi tendon organ occurs. The sensory efferent neuron of the Golgi tendon organ travels to the spinal cord and synapses with the alpha motoneuron of both the agonist muscle that it is monitoring and the antagonistic muscle. Inhibition of the agonist muscle and its synergists along with facilitation of the antagonists occurs, thereby relieving the tension. The harmful tension within the muscle is alleviated and potential damage to the musculotendinous unit avoided.

This protective mechanism of the Golgi tendon organs can be modified and potentially overridden. It may be possible to disinhibit the effects of the Golgi tendon organs and thereby raise the level of inhibition. This possibility may explain some of the injuries experienced by highly trained athletes who train with maximal weight training.

Proprioceptive Contribution Debate

Before the 1970s, articular receptors in the joint capsule were held primarily responsible for joint proprioception (Schulte & Happel, 1990). Since then there has been considerable debate as to whether muscular and articular mechanoreceptors interact. It has also been demonstrated that contraction of the muscular unit with either joint angle change or increased muscular tension plays a significant role in conscious joint proprioception (Cross & McCloskey, 1973; Goodwin, McCloskey, & Matthews, 1972). Miller has suggested that one of the functions of the muscle in the proprioceptive mechanism may be the modulation of joint afferent discharge (Miller, 1973). Many tendons insert or communicate directly with the joint capsule, and certain muscles such as the articularis genu and articularis cubiti seem to be specifically designed to generate periarticular tissue changes (Rowinski, 1990). These findings seem to demonstrate that mechanoreceptor modulation by muscular tension is readily apparent and possibly very important to the overall physiologic mechanoreceptor mechanism.

Dykes (1984) has proposed a concept of the sensory mechanoreceptors representing a continuum rather than separate distinct classes. This concept is further illustrated by research that demonstrated a relationship between the muscle spindle sensory afferent and the joint mechanoreceptors (Cafarelli & Bigland, 1979). McCloskey has also demonstrated a relationship between the cutaneous afferent and the joint mechanoreceptors (McCloskey, 1978). These studies suggest a complex role for the joint mechanoreceptors in coordinated controlled movement.

Information generated and encoded by the mechanoreceptors in the muscle tendon units are projected upward in the CNS to the cortex (Phillips, Powell, & Wiesendanger, 1971). Articular joint mechanoreceptors project upward in the CNS to the cerebellum by three separate spinal pathways (Haddad, 1953). How this information is utilized in producing smooth controlled movement is unknown at this time. Knowledge of the basic physiology of how these muscular and joint mechanoreceptors

work together in the production of smooth controlled coordinated motion is critical in developing a rehabilitation training program. Understanding these relationships and functional implications will allow the program coordinator greater variability and success in returning athletes safely to their playing environment.

◆ Historical Perspective

Following Sherrington's introduction of the concept, proprioception received little attention in the medical literature until Palmer (1958) mentioned two brief references to the concept of sensory input originating from the mechanoreceptors. Research demonstrated reflexive muscle firing of the vastus medialis, semimembranosus, and sartorius muscles in anesthetized cats who had their medial collateral ligament stretched. Palmer then coined the concept of "ligamentomuscular reflex." Since that time, numerous papers have documented the importance of the mechanoreceptors in supraspinal activity.

An important study by Ekholm, Ekland, and Skoglund (1960) documented the activation of sensory reflexes by stimulation of the cat's medial collateral ligament. Their study showed the presence of receptors in the ligament as well as in the joint capsule. Baxendale and Ferrell (1980, 1982) later demonstrated that this reflex could be obliterated with a local anesthetic.

Kennedy, Alexander, and Hayes (1982), de Andrade, Grant, and Dixon (1965), and Spencer, Hayes, and Alexander (1984) documented reflexive inhibition of the quadriceps musculature with knee joint effusion. Freeman and Wyke (1967a) demonstrated the influence of joint mechanoreceptors on motor control by cutting the medial and posterior articular nerves in the knee joints of cats. Motor performance was then reassessed one year later. At the time of reassessment, significant alterations in motor reflexes were noted and, in some cases, the animals were unable to perform the motor test entirely.

While some of the research may be contradictory, all of the studies demonstrated the neurosensory role of the mechanoreceptors in the joint capsule and corresponding ligaments. Stimulation of these mechanoreceptors can cause muscle activity to occur, and the loss of sensory function can impair motor control patterns.

Freeman and Wyke (1967) suggested that the joint mechanoreceptors play a significant role in the normal reflex coordination of muscular tone utilized in posture and movement. They went on to speculate that these reflexes likely become disordered in the presence of capsular joint lesions. Gray (1978) described the use of an ankle disc in the rehabilitation of ankle injuries. The ankle disc proved valuable in the reeducation of the proprioceptive mechanoreceptors. Gray theorized that the likelihood of ankle twists may be increased by the lack of ankle position sense at the time of injury rather than by muscle weakness. Glencross and Thornton (1981) stated that the normal functioning of the joint and skilled actions is likely inadequate because of the distortion of proprioceptive signals. Therefore, rehabilitative techniques should be directed toward the improvement of neuromuscular coordination and kinesthetic awareness.

While the concept and value of proprioceptive mechanoreceptors have been documented in the literature, treatment techniques directed at improving their function generally have not been incorporated into the overall rehabilitative program. Gray (1986, 1990) has done an excellent job of educating individuals about the importance of functional exercise; however, the neurosensory function of the pericapsular structures has taken a backseat to the mechanical structural role. This is mainly a consequence of the lack of information about how the mechanoreceptors contribute to the specific functional activities (Gandevia & McCloskey, 1976). It has been very difficult to demonstrate any consistent variation in joint proprioception or kinesthetic awareness secondary to injury. This is likely due to the lack of objective clinical testing for normal versus abnormal. Alteration in joint proprioception secondary to injury may be related to either direct or indirect injury. Direct trauma effects would include disruption of the joint capsule or ligaments, whereas indirect effects can be illustrated by posttraumatic joint effusion or hemarthrosis. Even more unclear is

how surgical and nonsurgical interventions may facilitate the restoration of the neurosensory roles (Woo & Buckwater, 1987). Research should be directed toward developing new techniques to improve proprioception. In addition, due to sensory cutaneous input affecting and facilitating afferent signals from the muscular and joint receptors, work should also be undertaken toward designing more effective, less bulky braces to take advantage of the physiological phenomena (Woo & Buckwater, 1987).

Functional Implications

As we have learned, the afferent mechanoreceptors contribute to the CNS in several distinct capacities. In the simplest mechanism, the afferent fibers of the mechanoreceptor synapse with the spinal interneurons and produce reflexive facilitation or inhibition of the motor neurons (see Figure 2.1). This mechanism is responsible for regulating motor control of the antagonistic and synergistic patterns of muscular contraction. The next mechanism is the interaction with the vestibular system for control or facilitation of postural and equilibrium maintenance. Afferent mechanoreceptor input is important in the control of coordinated movement patterns.

Afferent mechanoreceptor input also works in concert with the muscle spindle complex by inhibiting antagonist muscle activity under conditions of rapid lengthening and periarticular distortion, both of which accompany postural disruption (Rowinski, 1990). In conditions of disequilibrium where simultaneous neural input exists, a neural pattern is generated that affects the muscular stabilizers, thereby returning equilibrium to the body's center of gravity.

At the highest level of contribution to the CNS is the ability of the mechanoreceptors to interact and influence cognitive awareness of body position and movement (Rowinski, 1990). The role of the mechanoreceptors in providing joint perception involves

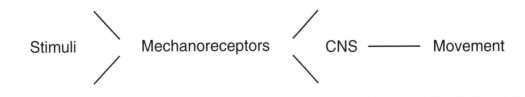

Figure 2.1   Direct synapse between mechanoreceptors and spinal interneurons that facilitates or inhibits motoneurons responsible for regulating movement.

their contribution to the feeling of deep pressure experienced at the limits of the joint's range of motion (Burgess, 1982). This could explain why there is very little receptor activity in the midrange of motion. Some research has indicated that the mechanoreceptors play no role in proprioceptive awareness. Goodwin, McCloskey, and Matthews (1972) and Matthews (1982) displayed no reduction in joint position sense following local anesthesia of the joint tissues. In addition, Griggs, Finerman, and Riley (1973) demonstrated little disruption in kinesthetic awareness following joint replacement surgery in humans in whom most of the joint receptors were surgically removed. The reason that each investigator may not have affected proprioceptive awareness may lie in the possibility that the muscle spindle is the important afferent in controlling position sense (Eklund, 1972; Goodwin et al., 1972; Matthews, 1982). The mechanoreceptors found near the joint may assist the muscle spindle in supplying information to the CNS. All of the afferent mechanoreceptors work together to supply information to the CNS, thereby affecting position sense. Kennedy and his associates (1982) demonstrated a loss of reflexive muscle splinting via posttraumatic mechanoreceptor discharge. This suggests that the dynamic stabilization process of co-contraction about the joint may be inhibited due to abnormal firing of

the afferent mechanoreceptors. The result would be an increased chance for reinjury due to the reflexive destabilization.

Open Versus Closed Kinetic-Chain Rehabilitation

Open-chain versus closed-chain rehabilitation typically refers to the status of the end segment of the extremity (see Figures 2.2a and 2.2b). In the case of the lower extremity, the foot would be fixed to the ground in closed-chain function. Traditional rehabilitation has always been performed in the open chain position with the proximal segment of the joint fixed with movement occurring distal to the axis of motion. The end segment is free, and movement is usually isolated to one of the three cardinal planes. Open-chain exercise is primarily a self-directed activity or action that is performed until muscle failure occurs. In this position, the musculoskeletal load created is abnormal in respect to function. This abnormal load is typically controlled via concentric or, less often, isometric muscle contractions that are inconsistent with normal joint motion. In regard to objective analysis, functional closed-chain exercise leads to increased isokinetic scores, whereas open-chain isokinetic exercise does not lead to increased functional performance scores.

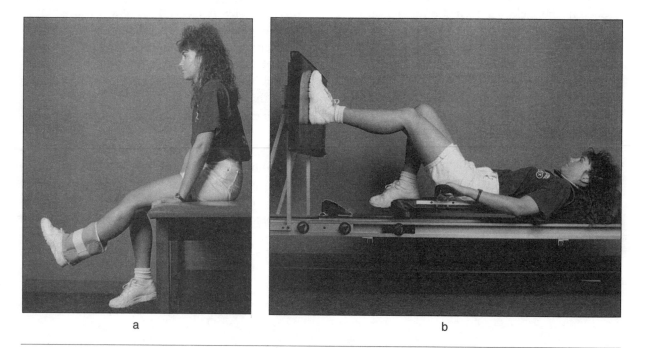

a   b

Figure 2.2 (a) Open-chain knee extension in which the distal segment is free to move. (b) Closed-chain knee extension in which the distal segment is fixed.

The importance of afferent mechanoreceptor input has already been discussed. From there, it does not take long to build a case for rehabilitating the individual in the closed-chain or functional weight-bearing position. Training in the closed-chain position facilitates normal proprioceptive feedback from the afferent mechanoreceptors. Exercise in the traditional open-chain position may foster inappropriate feedback to the CNS due to the difference in arthrokinematics. Joint play movements of rolling, gliding, and sliding are opposite each other in the open- and closed-chain positions. Enhancement of these proprioceptive feedback mechanisms in a weight-bearing position has a high degree of carryover and reinforces normal functional activity.

Closed-chain weight-bearing exercise is required to stimulate some of the mechanoreceptors found near the joint. Because Ruffini endings are located in the regions of greatest capsular stress and are sensitive to intracapsular fluid pressure changes, exercise in the normal weight-bearing position is required for normal physiologic stimulation. Pacinian corpuscles rapidly adapt and are active only at the onset of joint motion when sudden changes in joint movement and stress occur. Golgi-Mazzoni corpuscles are sensitive only to compression of the joint capsule in the plane perpendicular to the inner surface. This would require perpendicular axial loading for facilitation of these mechanoreceptors.

Gray, one of a few clinicians who address closed-chain function as it relates to the rehabilitation program, (1990) has done an excellent job in outlining the primary differences between open- and closed-chain function. Biomechanical research by Markolf, Bargar, Shoemaker, and Amstutz (1981) and Henning, Lynch, and Glick (1985) suggests that early closed-chain rehabilitative exercise is physiologically safe and less stressful than open-chain techniques. Biomechanical forces that are consistent with the early return to activity can be recreated safely in the closed-chain position.

With closed-chain training, the distal segment is fixed and movement occurs on both sides of the axis of motion. Movement in the closed-chain position is more functional in that motion can occur in all three planes, which is consistent with joint motion (see Figure 2.2b). Agonist, antagonist, and synergistic muscle groups can be activated concentrically, isometrically, or eccentrically to control normal physiologic loads associated with acceleration, deceleration, or stabilization of the joint in the weight-bearing position. The ability to train at variable velocities is consistent with normal acceleration and deceleration of the body, whereas in open-chain isotonic and isokinetic rehabilitation the velocity of the movement is controlled and predetermined.

Closed-chain rehabilitative techniques provide unlimited potential in the recreation of normal biomechanical stress-strain of functional activity. Performance of closed-chain rehabilitative techniques requires not only the self-directed action but also the reflexive reaction to changes in body position or equilibrium. Functional activities are performed until biomechanical or muscular substitution occurs.

♦ Balance and Kinesthetic Awareness

More than 100 years ago, Rhomberg observed and described postural and equilibrium deviations in a standing patient, which suggested musculoskeletal pathology. Since that time, clinicians have attempted objectively to measure and analyze postural instability that often accompanies neuromuscular pathology. The measure of body sway provides an index of postural stability.

Standing Balance

Standing balance represents a complex process that attempts to maintain postural equilibrium. Balance is maintained through a complex motor control task that requires integration of the afferent sensory mechanoreceptor information, neural processing within the CNS, and execution of the appropriate musculoskeletal responses. The basic concept of balance is the dynamic positioning of the body's center of gravity within the base of support in a given sensory environment. For example, in normal standing position, the center of gravity is centered over the feet. In an erect sitting position, the center of gravity is over the buttocks. Being able to stand upright is not a measure of balance. Individuals with fused or ankylosed joints can stand upright; however, they cannot adapt to change in the environment.

When an individual's center of gravity extends beyond the base of support, he or she has exceeded the limits of stability (defined as the outermost range in any direction that a person can lean from the vertical position without changing the original base of support). When the limits of stability are exceeded, a corrective step or stumble is required to prevent a fall. Balance therefore requires both neuromuscular coordination and adaptation.

The body of an apparently motionless standing individual undergoes continuous subconscious postural sway. These compensatory movements, side to side and front to back, help to maintain posture through complex reflexive mechanisms within the CNS. When postural equilibrium is disturbed, afferent reflexive contractions in the muscles help to restore balance. This reflexive muscle contraction causes a continuous postural sway that maintains the dynamic equilibrium of upright posture. ·

Maintaining balance requires an awareness of the body's center of gravity in relation to space and the ability to make appropriate musculoskeletal responses to control the body's mass. Traditionally, balance has been graded "good" if an individual can minimize postural sway and execute coordinated movement patterns upon movement of the support base. A balance disorder can be caused either by inaccurate afferent sensory orientation information or by inadequate muscle strength. Either of these conditions or a combination of the two can decrease ability to respond effectively when faced with disequilibrium. Because the ability to balance and maintain postural stability is critical to the acquisition or reacquisition of complex motor skills, it is very important to objectively quantify and rehabilitate equilibrium disorders.

Someone attempting to maintain equilibrium within his or her limits of stability will sway back and forth, creating a sway envelope. The midpoint of this envelope is the center of gravity alignment. When standing, your center of gravity is in the abdomen in the region of the lumbar vertebrae four. The exact location depends on body position. The sway envelope always lies within the individual's limits of stability. In the normal standing position, the center of gravity should also coincide with the center of limits of stability.

The limits of stability are approximately the same for everyone regardless of body height, because foot length also affects the limits. Foot length and height are directly related. Therefore, the resultant limits of stability remain fairly constant. The anterior-posterior (AP) limits of stability are ap-

proximately 12 degrees from the backward-most to forward-most position: 8 degrees forward and 4 degrees backward from the neutral position. The lateral limits of stability are directly related to the base of support width or stance width and height. With 4 inches between the feet, the lateral limits of support are approximately 16 degrees from side to side (8 degrees in either direction). If someone's center of gravity alignment coincides with the center of his or her limits of stability, the sway envelope for this person can be as large as 12 degrees AP and 16 degrees lateral, which is consistent with the limits of stability. If for some reason the center of gravity alignment is located off-center the limits of stability, a smaller sway envelope results. Disruption of balance is much more likely in this case as small sway oscillations are sufficient to push the center of gravity past the limits of stability.

Biomechanically, the limits of stability are similar for balance while standing and while walking. Standing in place may produce small shifts in the center of gravity from side to side and front to back. During normal ambulation, the center of gravity moves forward in a smooth coordinated fashion. During heel strike, the center of gravity is positioned at the back of the stability limits. With forward propulsion, the center moves to the front and is eventually pushed beyond the limits of stability, which causes the walker to step out with the other foot to avoid falling. As the body weight shifts to the opposite lower extremity, the limits of stability are reestablished and the process repeated.

With musculoskeletal dysfunction, either the limits of stability or the center of gravity alignment can change. Muscular weakness in the lower extremities or a decrease in the range of motion can shrink the limits of stability and place the person at increased risk for further injury or reinjury. This is due to the smaller sway envelope in which the individual balances. If the muscular weakness or decrease in range of motion is unilateral, the limits of stability will reduce toward the involved side.

Balance Disruption

In the event of disrupted balance, the body corrects itself (returns the center of gravity to a position within the limits of stability) in a variety of ways. Because the hip, knee, and ankle joints all lie between the center of gravity and the base of support, their afferent mechanoreceptor input can be used to control and improve balance. The response to balance disruption is primarily reflexive and automatic. The response is in a class of functionally organized long-loop responses that activate muscles to bring the body's center of gravity into a state of equilibrium. The sensory environment dictates the automatic postural response. These automatic postural reactions to disequilibrium occur before volition can be initiated and are not modified or controlled consciously. Although the primary strategies to control disrupted balance occur in the lower extremity, they are not limited exclusively to these joints. When faced with sudden disequilibrium or loss of balance, a person may reach out to grab a fixed object for added support.

The automatic postural responses used to correct anteroposterior body sway center on these possible strategies: ankle, hip, stepping, or combinations of these three (Horack & Washer, 1986; Nasher & McCollum, 1985).

Ankle Strategy

The ankle strategy requires correction of the center of gravity with slow, small movements. The body moves as a relatively rigid mass about the fixed ankle joints. The way muscle activates in the ankle strategy is opposite to the way it activates in the hip strategy. With backward sway, the anterior tibialis, quadriceps, and abdominal musculature contract to control the movement. To be effective, these muscular contractions must occur at equal strength in the correct distal to proximal sequence. If the timing of the contractions is disrupted, the postural reflex will fail in controlling the body's center of gravity. In anterior or forward sway, the gastrocmenius, hamstring, and paravertebral musculature all contract to prevent or control the sway. The head, hips, and ankles all move in phase with one another. This strategy is most effective when the center of gravity alignment is centered closely within the limits of stability and the body sway is relatively slow. When the center of gravity alignment is located outward, near the limits of stability, or when the body sway is much more rapid, the amount of muscular torque required to overcome the disruptive force greatly increases. In this example, the problem of controlling body sway with the ankle strategy is not due to inadequate muscle strength about the ankles but rather to the decreased lever arm length of the feet. When large muscular forces are applied to the feet, the heels lift off of the ground (calf raise). Here, to

prevent a fall, a fast correction strategy is required that does not utilize the ankle musculature. The hip strategy can fulfill that need.

Hip Strategy

In the hip strategy, the center of gravity is moved quickly over a short distance. The movement is centered in the hips as the feet exert force against the ground. Backward sway is controlled via the muscular forces of the paravertebral and hamstring musculature with some involvement of the gastrocnemius. Forward disruption is controlled by the abdominal and quadriceps muscles, and sometimes by the anterior tibialis. With the hip strategy, the head, hips, and ankles all move out of phase in relation to one another. In the case of rapid balance disruption, the limits of stability are reduced to only a few degrees. As a result, the individual is dangerously close to exceeding the limits. The hip strategy can produce a rapid contraction within the reduced sway envelope but cannot maintain or hold an offset center of gravity. As soon as the hips stop accelerating, the ground reaction forces disappear. Therefore, the force required to hold the offset center of gravity must come from the ankle strategy. Both the ankle and hip strategies require adequate range of motion and muscular strength about the joints. Additionally, the individual must be standing on a firm surface and possess the ability to sense the base of support.

Stepping Strategy

When the center of gravity is rapidly displaced or is displaced beyond the limits of stability, a stepping strategy is necessary to regain the body's equilibrium. In both cases, neither of the two other automatic postural strategies can generate enough force to control the center of gravity and move it back within the limits of stability. Consequently, a stepping strategy is needed to establish a new set of limits.

◆ Summary

We can see that balance is a complex process involving the integration of biomechanical, neurological sensory afferent, and muscular forces. This chapter has attempted to present the physiological foundations of motor learning with mechanoreceptor input to central processing. This proprioceptive or somatosensory information is one of the important components of balance. Those who display a decreased sense of balance may lack either the appropriate or sufficient quantity of afferent mechanoreceptor orientation information. In addition, muscular weakness may limit the ability to generate an effective correction response when faced with disequilibrium. In either case, the rehabilitation program must be adaptable and include functional exercise that incorporates balance and proprioceptive training to prepare the individual for return to activity. Failure to address this area will result in incomplete rehabilitation and possibly reinjury upon the athlete's return to function. The following chapters will build on this foundation of neurophysiological principles and apply the concepts practically.

CHAPTER 3

◆◆◆

Functional Testing

If you've read the first two chapters, you understand that functional progression needs to be included in your rehabilitation program. You know that the main purpose of functional progression is to ready an athlete for return to competition. In the traditional functional progression program, skills are performed, assessed, and progressed as a person tolerates. Individual skills are assessed to determine if the athlete can proceed in the functional progression program.

However, functional progression drills can also be used as tools to *assess* an athlete's function. *Functional testing* uses components of a functional progression program solely for the purpose of assessing that given function. In this chapter, you will learn to modify functional progression drills to serve as functional testing. You will also learn when functional testing should be performed; the relationship between functional testing, functional training, and functional progression; and the proper way to progress functional testing evaluations.

◆ Functional Testing Versus Functional Progression

Perhaps the best way to illustrate the difference between functional progression and functional testing is to contrast the desired results of the two activities. Functional progression is a series of sport-specific movement patterns progressed according to the athlete's tolerance. The desired effect of functional progression is a timely and safe return to sport.

Functional testing, on the other hand, breaks function down for the purpose of assessing that function. Functional testing is a one-time, maximal effort that is performed to assess performance.

Functional progression activities and functional testing sometimes overlap. Some functional testing drills may be components of the functional progression program. Let's use a specific drill as an example.

Step-ups (see page 11) are an integral component of the functional progression program following a lower extremity injury. Step-ups encourage weight bearing and weight shifting, and are also a good strengthening exercise. They help prepare healing tissue to accept the demands of an athlete's return to sport. Step-ups also can be used as a functional test. Having the athlete do repetitive step-ups to determine endurance allows you to compare performance to preinjury level or to the function of noninjured teammates.

◆ Functional Testing Versus Functional Training

Another area that needs to be differentiated from functional testing is *functional training*. Functional training is the repeated performance of an athletic skill, solely for the purpose of perfecting that skill. When you think of a typical team practice setting, the concept of functional training makes sense. Day after day the athlete practices, repeating the same basic skills. The coaches hope that repeated performance of the skill will make the skill automatic for the athlete.

Again, there can be some overlap between functional training and functional progression. As an example, let's use one-legged hopping. One-legged hopping on the injured lower extremity is a skill stressed in the training of jumpers. Hopping on one leg is an excellent way to develop strength, power, agility, and foot quickness. However, one-legged hopping is also an ideal functional test to determine the individual's willingness to accept weight on the involved leg after injury.

In functional training, one-legged hopping is used to improve sport-specific function. In functional testing, one-legged hopping is used to evaluate the athlete's performance of this one specific skill. As you can see, functional testing lies somewhere between functional progression and functional training. Functional testing is a two-way street with overlap between functional progression and functional training. While sharing many similarities with functional progression and training, functional testing remains unique.

◆ Why Perform Functional Testing?

Performance of a sport-specific skill means more to the athlete than many of the tests traditionally used in the formal rehabilitation setting. Consequently, functional testing evaluates performance in a purposeful manner. In addition to providing yourself and the athlete with meaningful feedback, functional testing can be used to qualify team norms and give the athlete psychological reassurance. Let's examine the reasons that you should incorporate functional testing into your rehabilitation program.

Assessing Sport and Position Function

Why is it necessary to assess sport function via functional testing? Speed, strength, agility, and power are all vital components to many sports. All of these are easily assessed by conventional means. Speed can be measured with a stopwatch, strength can be evaluated through weight lifting, and agility can be assessed with simple balance tests. But only when you combine all of these components are you able to assess function.

So, functional testing is performed to assess sport-specific function. To determine sport-specific function, the athlete's sport-specific skills need to be assessed. But function within a specific sport needs to be qualified, as does the function of each specific position in the sport. Take our previous example of American football. Function of an offensive back is far different from that of an offensive lineman. The offensive back position

requires speed, agility, quick acceleration and deceleration, and hand-eye coordination. In contrast, the offensive lineman requires greater strength than the back must have. Functional testing breaks down the athlete's function in his or her sport and then provides a way to qualify that function.

A good functional test for the offensive back may be repetitive single-leg step-ups, whereas the lineman may be better served by performing mini-squats. These skills were described as functional progression tools in chapter 1 but will be explained as testing tools later in this chapter.

Qualifying Function for Team Norms

Another reason to perform functional testing is to establish team norms. Each athlete required to perform a function must possess intrinsic skills that are prerequisites for successful performance of the skill. To identify the functions an athlete must fulfill in a given sport, you need to break down sport-specific and position-specific skills. Functional testing will assist you in establishing team norms for a given function.

Let's use volleyball to help illustrate functional testing for team norms. As you will see on page 41, vertical jump assessment is an excellent functional test and invaluable in establishing team norms. In the case of functional testing, the vertical jump can be easily measured for all team members by recording the distances that each member jumps and then standardizing the jumps for height. Norms can then be established for the entire team. These normative values are especially helpful as motivational tools in the training and rehabilitation program.

Assessing Function During Rehabilitation

For the rehabilitation professional, perhaps the most meaningful role functional testing plays is in the assessment of function during rehabilitation. An athlete's accomplishment of clinic-based goals such as adequate range of motion, strength, and endurance is not enough for you to return the athlete to sport. That is the very reason for functional progression. However, certain functional tests performed at the right time during rehabilitation are helpful complements to functional progression.

To what extent has the importance of functional testing been recognized? Well, the International

Knee Documentation Committee added a functional test to their recommended battery of tests following anterior cruciate ligament reconstruction (Magee, 1992). The test that this group of noted knee authorities has adopted is a single-leg hop for distance and is discussed on page 40.

Athletes can work single-plane knee extension on an isokinetic machine, but until actual function is stressed, you have no idea how they are really doing in terms of progress toward returning to the playing field. Functional testing can be helpful in this regard. By starting with simple and progressing to more complex functional tests, both you and the athlete can get an accurate idea of the athlete's readiness for competition.

Providing Psychological Reassurance of Function

Usually, at some point in the rehabilitation program the athlete grows tired of the purely clinical approach. This is one reason that the program should be varied. Yes, rehabilitation should be taxing for the athlete, but it should also be enjoyable. But no matter how much you vary a program, clinic-based rehabilitation can become monotonous. The athlete may have difficulty connecting progress in the clinic with progress toward returning to sport. At this juncture, functional testing can be used as a dose of reality for the athlete. If the athlete can see that his or her vertical jump was 12 inches 2 weeks ago and that this week it has increased to 14 inches, then clinic-based rehabilitation achieves credibility for him or her.

On the other hand, there may also come a point during rehab that the athlete sees function as better than it really is. For example, an athlete who readily handles the clinic-based program may believe that he or she is prepared to return to the playing field. Again, at this point functional testing can serve as a reality check. When the athlete first tries to jump as far as possible from the involved leg and land solely on the involved side, he or she might have second thoughts about being game ready.

♦ When Should Functional Testing Be Performed?

Now that you know why functional testing is beneficial for you and your athletes, let's discuss timing. Generally speaking, functional testing should be performed

- during preseason screening,
- during rehabilitation, and
- immediately after injury.

During Preseason Screening

If preseason screening is done at all, far too often it is not sport-specific or as comprehensive as it should be. A good preseason screening program should include a variety of sport-specific functional tests. Jumping sports should include jumping and hopping tests, endurance sports should stress endurance, and strength sports should include strength assessment. Functional tests can be used to assess these along with other functions.

By requiring sport-specific functional tests before the season, you can establish team norms and take corrective measures with individuals whose values fall below the norms. Also, should an athlete be injured during the season, preinjury functional test values are useful in setting rehabilitation goals.

During Rehabilitation

As we've discussed, rehabilitation professionals will find functional testing most beneficial during the formal rehabilitation program. Many authors have noted ligamentous instability, lower-quarter muscular weakness, patellofemoral symptoms, and other signs and symptoms following injury to the anterior cruciate ligament. Some parameters correlate with decreased functional testing results, and some do not (Barber, Noyes, Mangine, McCloskey, & Hartman, 1990; Friden, Zatterstrom, Lindstrand, & Moritz, 1990; Gauffin, Pettersson, Tegner, & Tropp, 1990; Gauffin, Pettersson, & Tropp, 1990; Tegner, Lysholm, Lysholm, & Gillquist, 1986.). Therefore, to correlate formal rehabilitation with functional capabilities, functional testing is a must. The peak torque generated on an isokinetic unit can serve as a guideline for activity, but the best test to determine if an athlete is ready to perform more functional skills is through functional testing. However, Paine (personal conversation) did find a correlation between isokinetic knee extension values at 60 degrees/second and single-leg hop for distance, but he found no correlation at 240 degrees/second.

Along with providing an accurate objective feedback tool during rehabilitation, functional testing can serve as a positive or negative psychological reinforcement to the patient. When the athlete doubts his or her progress or questions if traditional rehabilitation efforts are paying off, functional testing can be conducted to demonstrate progress to the individual. On the other hand, if an athlete then questions why traditional efforts must be continued, or believes that no further rehabilitation is needed, functional testing can be used to document existing deficits.

Immediately After Injury

Functional testing can also be of help immediately after injury. Certainly, many clinic-based therapists may never be responsible for evaluating or treating acute sport injury; however, functional testing performed immediately after injury helps to identify the injury and provides a good prognostic tool. Perhaps the functional classification of ankle sprains proposed by Jackson, Ashley, and Powell (1974) illustrates this best. In Table 3.1 you can see that instead of classifying ankle sprain according to the amount of joint laxity, injury is classified according to the athlete's ability to function—that is, the extent of ability to raise up on the toes. This simple assessment is much easier to perform than trying to assess ligamentous laxity after pain, swelling, and reflex inhibition sets in. If you are able to classify function immediately after injury, you will be able to estimate the degree of severity and set realistic rehabilitation goals.

♦ Progression of Functional Testing

As we have seen, functional testing shares similarities with functional progression drills. As in the case of functional progression, skills to be functionally tested are introduced into the formal rehabilitation program as soon as the athlete is ready. Adequate strength, range of motion, and other prerequisites for functional progression also apply to functional testing.

When you need to assess primary skills that the athlete will require to function on the playing field, you need to do so in a safe manner. Similar to functional progression drills, functional testing activities are progressed from simple to complex. Although the functional test may be a one-time assessment, if the demands of that assessment are too great for the healing tissue to accept, reinjury may result.

Because virtually all sport activities involve closed-chain lower extremity function, functional testing should be performed in the closed kinetic chain. However, range of motion, movement speed, and additional resistance for testing may be more easily controlled in the open chain. Therefore, adequate, safe function in an open chain may be the first step of functional testing.

As an example, let's use an injured basketball player with patellar tendinitis. Eccentric loads placed on connective tissue have been shown to load tendon tissue greater than muscle fiber (Doss & Karpovich, 1965; Stanish, Rubinovich, & Curwin, 1986; Stauber, 1989). This is easily demonstrated by the fact that most jumping athletes with patellar tendinitis will complain of greatest pain not when taking off from a jump (concentric quadriceps contraction) but when landing (eccentric quadriceps contraction). Therefore, eccentrics should figure highly in your program to stress the affected tissue. However, because of superimposed body weight, even the least stressful closed-chain activities may increase pain. If this occurs, simple open-chain strengthening efforts should be stressed, with emphasis on controlled eccentric contractions. The same principles apply in open- and closed-chain testing procedures. As you well know, rehabilitation is not black and white. Even with excellent clinical research, there remains a good deal of gray.

Table 3.1 Jackson's Functional Classification of Ankle Sprain

Mild sprain	Moderate sprain	Severe sprain
No limp	Limp	Prefers crutches for weight bearing
Difficulty hopping symmetrically on injured ankle	Inability to raise up on toes or hop on injured ankle	

Remember this when you are trying to decide on open- or closed-chain assessment and rehabilitation techniques.

Bilateral Support Tests

Once controlled, open-chain activities are tolerated, proceed to closed-chain tests. Weight bearing on both legs or arms is easier than single-leg or single-arm weight bearing. Functional testing should begin with bilateral support drills—drills performed with both legs or both arms supported. After a lower extremity injury, stress mini-squats. After an upper extremity injury, stress weight bearing in a hands-and-knees position or a modified push-up position. To assess function in these positions, let's first look at lower extremity function and then address the upper extremity.

Lower Extremity

Mini-squats are discussed in detail on page 10. Whether done for functional testing or functional progression, the exercise is performed in the same manner. To use any functional progression drill for assessment, the function must be either qualified or quantified. As the mini-squat is a stationary activity, you can't use distance to qualify function. Instead, use time to quantify function. In the case of mini-squats, the athlete is asked either to perform as many squats as possible in a set amount of time or to hold a mini-squat in midrange. In both cases the chosen time should be sport specific. For example, you may have a gymnast hold for the amount of time that positions must be maintained on the balance beam, whereas the downhill skier should hold the position longer to approximate the time of a traditional downhill run. It works best to use a stopwatch, but any watch with a second hand will do.

When assessing mini-squats, observe closely to make sure undesired substitutions do not occur in place of the desired movement. When proper form breaks down, stop the clock. Frequent undesired substitutions include

- inadequate range of motion,
- poor symmetry, and
- unequal weight shift.

Inadequate range of motion. The athlete must consistently perform through a given arc of motion. To ensure proper motion is maintained throughout the mini-squat, pass a string beneath the athlete and make sure contact with the string is maintained the entire desired time, or for every repetition. (A string works better than a stool or a chair, as it is hard to monitor the amount of weight that is resting on the stool or chair.)

An excellent tool for accurate assessment of stationary, closed-chain testing activities is the RightWeigh.[1] This apparatus can be attached to the individual to monitor performance (see Figure 3.1). The athlete is asked to perform a given task at one cadence and through a given arc of motion set on the RightWeigh. Upon test completion, the RightWeigh provides scores based on the individual's ability to move at the preset pace and through the appropriate range of motion.

Poor symmetry. The athlete should perform the mini-squat with feet shoulder-width apart and toes

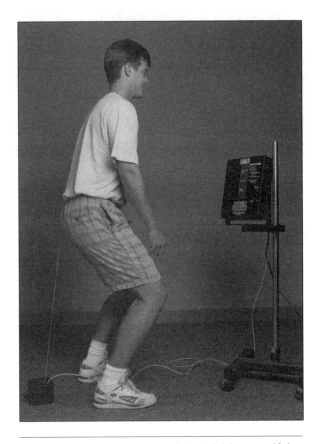

Figure 3.1 The RightWeigh is helpful in quantifying performance of open-chain or closed-chain rehabilitation testing or treatment activities.

---

[1]Baltimore Therapeutic Equipment, Baltimore, Maryland.

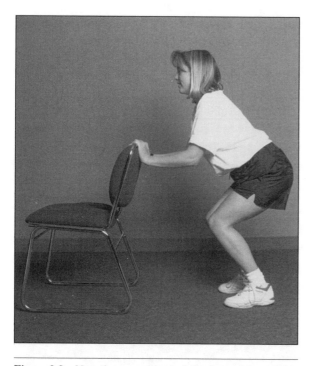

Figure 3.2 Note the excessive trunk flexion and the anterior slope of the tibia in this mini-squat substitution drill (lateral view).

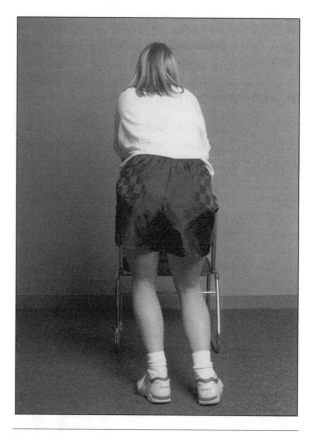

Figure 3.3 From behind the individual look for unequal weight shift over the noninvolved lower extremity.

pointing straight ahead. The buttocks should remain over the heels. The knees should stay behind the toes with the lower leg as close to perpendicular to the floor as possible. Common substitutions are excessive trunk flexion or lower legs too far forward (see Figure 3.2).

Unequal weight shift. Observe from behind to assure that the athlete's pelvis is parallel to the floor and the spine directly over the pelvis. Often, excessive lateral flexion over the noninvolved lower extremity occurs if the individual is substituting (see Figure 3.3).

Upper Extremity

Strength of the upper extremity after injury can be readily assessed through functional testing. Bilateral support drills on hands and knees or in a modified push-up (or wheelbarrow) position do not fully assess strength if elbows are locked. In this position, the wrist is stabilized on the floor and the olecranon fits snugly into the olecranon fossa. Therefore, functional assessment of the contractile tissue

is not maximized. As with the knee during mini-squats, the elbow must remain slightly flexed to allow for more muscle function to maintain the position.

The hands-and-knees position is certainly functional for a wrester or a football lineman, but its benefit is doubtful for other athletes. Another concern is that on hands and knees the arms are bearing only partial body weight. This is why the modified push-up position is used. Removing the knees from a supporting position puts more weight on the arms (see Figure 3.4a). Again, bilateral upper extremity support drills are stationary, so it's best to use time to measure function. Ask the athlete to maintain a modified push-up position for a sport-specific time. Or count the number of push-ups the athlete can perform. Another position that stresses the upper extremities is the standing push-up, which minimizes the effect of gravity and may be tolerated by the individual earlier in the testing sequence (see Figure 3.4b).

Observe carefully to guard against substitutions. Once substitution occurs, stop the test. Substitu-

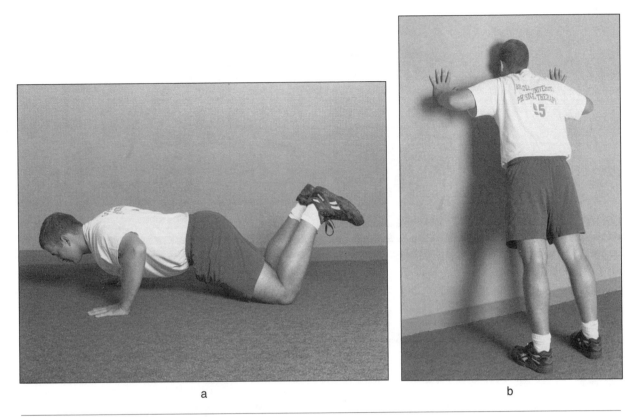

| a | b |

Figure 3.4 (a) Quadruped position. To assure appropriate, symmetrical weight bearing, the athlete bears weight through flexed knees, versus the toes with extended knees in the traditional push-up position. (b) Standing position wall push-up.

tions for bilateral upper extremity support drills are similar to those of the lower extremity.

Inadequate range of motion. If the athlete does not perform push-ups through the specified arc of motion, try passing a string or other suitable object under his or her chest (see Figure 3.5)

Poor symmetry. The arms should be maintained at shoulder's width. The upper arms should be held

at 90 degrees of abduction. Palms should be flat on the floor (a slight amount of ulnar deviation is acceptable; see Figure 3.6). The athlete should maintain the appropriate position for the duration of the midrange push-up, as well as for the repetitive push-ups.

Unequal weight shift. Observe the athlete from above to assure that proper weight distribution is

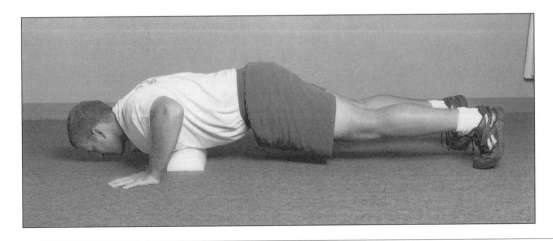

Figure 3.5 A suitable object can be passed under the individual's chest to assure consistent range of motion in the push-up.

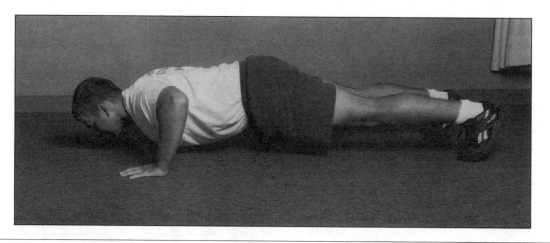

Figure 3.6 This position can be used as an early test to determine functional strength and the ability to accept weight symmetrically through the upper extremities.

maintained. To substitute for upper extremity weakness, the athlete will commonly shift laterally away from the involved side, which is demonstrated by an elevated contralateral hip (see Figure 3.7).

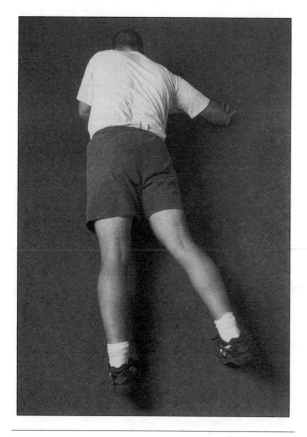

Figure 3.7 When watching for substitutions, look for excessive lateral trunk flexion away from the involved upper extremity and/or unequal hip height.

Unilateral Support Tests

After a lower extremity injury, a vital key to the functional progression program is the step-up. This is equally true for the functional testing sequence. A successful completion of step-ups eases physical and psychological concerns. The introductory chapter described step-ups in detail. In following chapters dealing with sport-specific functional progression programs, variations of step-ups will be emphasized. Here, your only concern with step-ups is in their usefulness as a functional testing tool. This versatile activity will be described as a functional test for lower extremity injury. A modification of it is also useful for upper extremity injury.

Lower Extremity

For functional testing, a standardized, uniform height must first be chosen. Typically, you'll use a height of 8 inches, but if your athletes are shorter or taller than average, make appropriate adjustments. Step-ups as a functional test are performed just as they are for functional progression. Because step-ups are stationary tests, time is the only way to qualify and quantify function. As with mini-squats, performance of step-ups can be expressed as either the length of time the athlete maintains a midrange step-up or as the number of step-ups completed in a set time. Because good balance is required for single-leg stance, if midrange contraction maintenance is used, you need to watch for substitutions to correct for loss of balance. As with bilateral support drills, sport-specific time frames should be considered. The RightWeigh is beneficial in quantifying and qualifying performance.

Substitutions that the athlete may use for properly performed step-ups are similar to those you see in mini-squats. Inadequate range of motion, inappropriate weight shift, poor symmetry, poor eccentric control, and the use of the contralateral plantar flexors may be demonstrated by athletes who are fatigued or unready to perform step-ups. An excessive height of step might also cause undesired substitutions.

Inadequate range of motion. When stressing repetitive step-ups, make sure that the athlete returns to touch the noninvolved heel to the ground after each step-up (see Figure 3.8). The step-up should be completed to a position of 5 to 10 degrees of knee flexion instead of extending the involved knee completely. Complete knee extension is usu-

ally easier for the individual and may stress the posterior capsule and other secondary restraints of the knee after injury. A deliberate, controlled step-up is a better assessment of strength and minimizes genu recurvatum.

Inappropriate weight shift. You'll need keen observation skills to ensure the athlete does not substitute. Internal rotation at the hip with an overall valgus attitude at the knee is accompanied by an excessive lateral shift toward the involved side best observed from behind the athlete.

Poor eccentric control. Inadequate strength for step-ups will be best demonstrated by poor eccentric control. As the athlete attempts to lower the noninvolved leg to the starting position, inadequate strength of the involved leg results in a quick, noncontrolled descent.

Use of contralateral plantar flexors. If the athlete is allowed to lower body weight onto the toes of

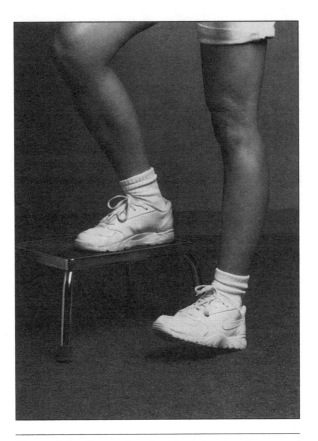

Figure 3.8 The noninvolved heel touches the ground between step-ups.

the weight-bearing noninvolved leg, the next step-up will be done with the assistance of the noninvolved leg's powerful plantar flexors. To prevent this, make sure the step-up always begins with the noninvolved leg bearing weight through the heel, keeping the midfoot and toes off the floor (see Figure 3.9).

Upper Extremity

Unilateral support tests for the arm are modifications of the 4-point weight-bearing or wheelbarrow positions. Repetitive one-armed push-ups or timed midrange positions can be performed the same as bilateral upper extremity support tests. One additional modification is the one-armed spin. This test involves bearing weight on the involved side only, as shown in Figure 3.10. Maintaining the arm and both feet as the only points of contact with the ground, the athlete spins about the fixed arm in either a clockwise or counterclockwise direction. Record the length of time it takes the athlete to complete a predetermined number of revolutions

around the arm. Another way to assess this function is to have the individual perform the maximum number of arm spins in a sport-specific amount of time. Though this skill assesses lower extremity function, it is primarily used to evaluate the function of the arm in providing support of the moving body.

◆ Bilateral and Unilateral Support Drills (Loaded)

If an athlete can tolerate bilateral but not unilateral support testing, loaded bilateral support drills may be the answer. In most cases, bilateral support tests will progress directly to unilateral tests. However, loaded bilateral support tests (with extra resistance) may occasionally be required prior to unilateral work. In such cases, the athlete simply performs the functional tests for maximum time held or for maximal repetitions in a given time with extra weight added to the body. Both legs are used for support, and extra weight can be added via a closed-

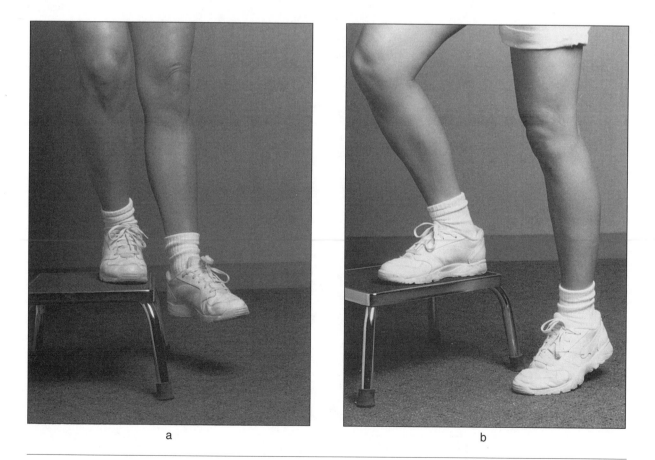

a   b

Figure 3.9   (a) Heel touch of contralateral lower extremity should be stressed. (b) Substitution by plantar flexing the ankle.

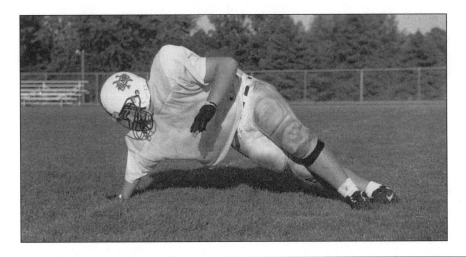

Figure 3.10 The weight of the body is accepted through the involved upper extremity as the individual spins clockwise and counterclockwise around the stationary arm.

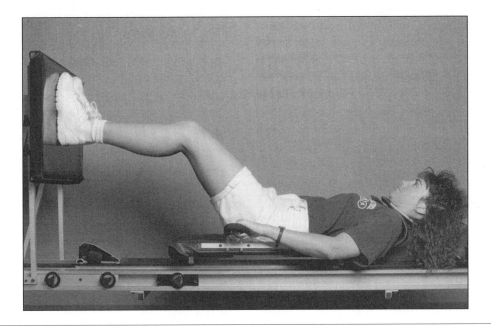

Figure 3.11 The Shuttle 2001 is an outstanding tool for functional testing of the lower quarter in a bilateral support or unilateral support manner.

chain leg press, a weighted vest, or on the Shuttle 2001[2] (see Figure 3.11). The extra weight should be a standard percentage of total body weight or lean body weight.

If unilateral support testing is not strenuous enough, the same principles can be applied for midrange or repetitive step-ups on the leg press or Shuttle 2001, with a weight vest, or with surgical tubing. Remember that you must keep the added resistance consistent if used in functional testing.

[2]Contemporary Design Company, Glacier, Washington.

♦ Bilateral and Unilateral Nonsupport Drills

Hopping (bilateral support) and jumping (unilateral support) tests are excellent ways to evaluate function. Along with step-ups, hopping and especially jumping will give you and your athletes a good idea of comparative lower extremity function. Up to now, we have discussed functional tests performed in a stationary position. Hopping and jumping can be assessed in a stationary position as well, but they can also be evaluated as the athlete performs a maximum jump or hop for vertical or horizontal distance.

Repetitive Jumping and Hopping for Time

Because jumping and hopping can be assessed in a stationary position, you can use time to qualify function. Repetitive jumps or hops can be performed for a predetermined, sport-specific length of time, with you recording the number of jumps or hops completed. Another option is to have the athlete perform a set number of jumps or hops and record how long it takes. When repetitive jumps or hops are performed for time, a sport-specific time should be used. This is especially helpful for wrestlers, boxers, and figure skaters, as well as for others who compete for specific durations.

These tests emphasize the amount of time the athlete can perform, but sometimes it is difficult to assure consistency throughout the testing. Observation and qualification of the height the athlete jumps or hops must also be factored into the assessment. Bench jumps or hops are often helpful in this area. When doing bench jumps, the athlete jumps side to side over a stationary object (a small bench or step stool, or a high-jump cross-bar on top of two cones may be used). A uniform percentage of the athlete's height will assure consistency when testing more than one person. The time it takes for the individual to do a set number of jumps, or the number of jumps performed in a sport-specific time frame can be used to qualify or quantify function. When appropriate, substitute hopping for jumping. Whether the athlete is jumping or hopping, safety should always be of prime importance.

Jumping and Hopping for Distance

Virtually all sports involve a component of power, and one of the best ways to assess function along with power is with jumping or hopping tests for distance. Distances can be assessed either horizontally or vertically. One-time maximal jumping off both feet or hopping off one foot can be tested as the individual leaps upward or forward. Now that an actual distance is your main concern, you

must be consistent and accurate in your measurements. Give careful attention to beginning and ending positions, as well as to substitution movement. Specifics regarding measuring vertical and horizontal jumps follow in their respective discussions.

Horizontal Hopping and Jumping for Distance

Horizontal and vertical jumping are good tools to develop team norms as a gauge of lower extremity strength and power. Especially beneficial in preseason screening, horizontal and vertical jumping can be performed by the entire team. Normative values can be calculated, and athletes who function below the norm can be given corrective measures. Horizontal and vertical hopping can also be used but are better for assessment in comparing one leg to the other. During rehabilitation, horizontal jumping provides an invaluable assessment of not only strength, power, and kinesthesia of the affected leg, but also of the athlete's willingness to accept weight and "trust" the leg. Maximum horizontal and vertical hopping, first off one leg and then the other, provides an easy side-to-side comparison of function.

When using horizontal jumping and hopping in functional testing, keep the following points in mind.

Function.   Let the athlete's specific task guide you in deciding whether to assess the athlete horizontally or vertically. Although vertical assessment is a fantastic measure of overall function, the horizontal component is just as important for certain athletes. For example, sprinters, hockey players, and basketball players all need to cover a horizontal playing surface quickly, so for these athletes, jumping or hopping horizontally should be stressed along with any vertical assessments.

Consistency in measuring.   The take-off and especially the landing position must be measured consistently. All clinicians differ in certain areas, and the measurement of functional tests may be no different. Strive to be consistent from test to test.

When assessing jumping or hopping for horizontal distance, keep these tips in mind:

• Use momentum consistently. Most tests are performed allowing the athlete to generate momentum in the stationary position by swinging the arms.

• When assessing hopping off one leg, make sure not to allow assistance from the opposite leg. Assistance from the opposite leg should not be allowed prior to take-off for balance or to assist in providing propulsion for the hop.

• Measure distances consistently. Standard measurement is usually from the back edge of the starting to the landing position of the heel.

Symmetry in movement. Try to ensure that weight shift and weight acceptance is consistent from leg to leg. As technology becomes more affordable, force plates are being used to help ensure symmetrical weight bearing at take-off and landing. A sophisticated system of force plates has been developed for this very purpose. The Fastex®[3] system is a group of integrated force plates interfaced with a computer for data analysis and storage. Used for both testing and training, the Fastex can measure static and dynamic weight acceptance as the athlete performs various maneuvers (see Figure 3.12).

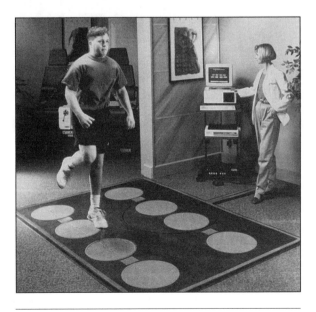

Figure 3.12 The computer interfaced force platform system is an excellent way to assess reaction time, mobility, and stability for a quantifiable functional test.

Vertical Hopping and Jumping for Distance

Basketball, volleyball, and other jumping athletes should routinely be tested for vertical hopping and jumping ability. These assessments are appropriate in the preseason as well as during rehabilitation.

As we've discussed, accurate and consistent measurement is of utmost importance when assessing vertical height functional testing. Measurements of both the starting position and the maximum height position must be consistent. Varied positions of ankle plantar flexion or scapular rotation are acceptable testing methods, but be aware of the inherent differences for each position used. Different philosophies are employed as to whether the athlete starts flat-footed or up on the toes and whether the arms are held out to the side or up overhead. It does not matter what your personal philosophy or rationale is, just be consistent. Maximum reach can be measured by putting chalk on the athlete's fingertips. The Vertec[4] is an outstanding tool to accurately record vertical jump performance (see Figure 3.13).

When you use horizontal or vertical jumping for side-to-side comparisons, deficits are expressed as a percentage of involved side to noninvolved side. To arrive at the percentage, simply divide the distance of the involved leg by the distance of the noninvolved leg and multiply the total by 100. For example, if the vertical jump off the right leg is 20 inches and the jump off the noninvolved left leg is 31 inches, the percent deficit would be figured this way:

$$20/31 \times 100 = 65\%$$

Just as functional progression must be sport specific, functional testing should be related to the athlete's sport. Different sports require different jumping patterns, so you need to make functional assessment sport specific for jumping. For example, when assessing vertical jump of a basketball forward, you may allow a one-step approach before jumping. But when assessing function of a volleyball hitter, you may wish to allow a three-step approach. As we move on to more aggressive testing methods, more movement of the individual is allowed. Let's progress to activities involving more complex movement patterns to assess more aggressive sport-specific function.

---

[3]Cybex, Ronkonkoma, New York.

[4]Sports Imports, Columbus, Ohio.

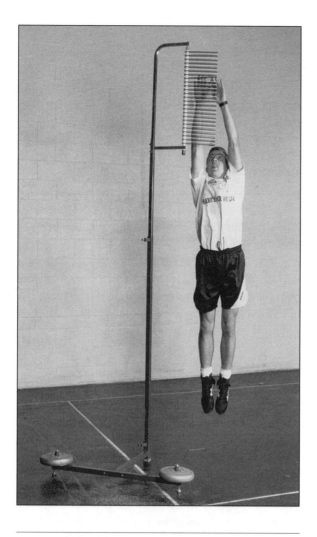

Figure 3.13   Vertec is a portable, accurate assessment tool that has become the standard for vertical jump functional testing. Starting position is noted and the athlete then jumps, striking the slats to mark the highest point of the jump.

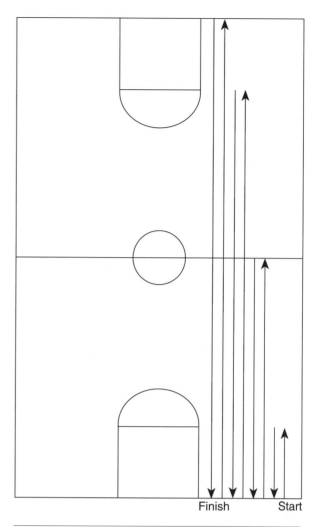

Finish   Start

Figure 3.14   The "suicide drill" is utilized for functional testing. Ensure that the athlete alternates legs in deceleration and pivoting. Distances covered should be sport specific.

◆ Agility Drills

Agility runs, combined with vertical or horizontal hopping or jumping, provide you with one of the best sport-specific tests available. These tests involve multiplane movements and stress-controlled acceleration, deceleration, cutting, and pivoting. As always, not every one of these tests will be applicable in every case. Choose the ones that meet your needs and modify the ones that do not.

Difficulty Shuttle Run

The simplest agility run involves straight plane running, deceleration, pivoting, and acceleration. You have no doubt seen this drill performed. The shuttle run, also known as suicide drills, up-and-

backs, or minute drills, are performed on a basketball court but can be modified for any playing surface. The athlete begins at the baseline, runs to the nearest free throw line, touches the line, and returns to the baseline. After touching the baseline, the athlete sprints to the half-court line, touches it, and sprints back to the baseline. The athlete then sprints to the far free throw line, returns to the baseline, sprints to the far baseline, and then finally sprints back to the starting baseline (see Figure 3.14).

Make sure the athlete touches the line each time. Also, when decelerating and pivoting to touch the line, the athlete should alternate feet. In other words, on the first pivot at the near free throw line and on the return trip to the baseline, the right foot should touch the line. Then after the trip to the half-court line, the left foot should touch the line. You can use variations of this test, depending on the sport. For example, an American-football lineman will not frequently be required to sprint the distance of a basketball court, so you may wish to set up a 10- or 20-yard test. Tennis players, American-football defensive backs, and other athletes who must sometimes run backward may require a similar test performed backward. Hockey players can do a similar drill on ice.

T-Drill Shuffle

An agility test that involves more lateral movement than the shuttle run is the T-drill shuffle. Using cones or other suitable markers, set up a T-shaped course at a sport-specific distance (usually 10 yards). Starting at marker A, the athlete sprints forward and stops abruptly at marker B. Pushing laterally off the planted right foot, the athlete then laterally shuffles left for 5 yards before stopping on the left foot at marker C. The athlete then laterally shuffles 10 yards to marker D. Here, the athlete pushes laterally off the right foot and shuffles back to center marker B, from where he or she then runs backward (backpedals) to the starting point (see Figure 3.15). This test is a must for individuals involved in sports requiring lateral movement.

T-Drill Cut

A combination of the suicide drill and the T-drill shuffle is the T-drill cut. A test course is set up as explained under the T-drill shuffle. This time the athlete sprints to marker B and side-shuffles left to marker C. Here the athlete pivots off the left foot and sprints right to marker D. At marker D, she or he pivots off the left foot, sprints to marker B, and then backpedals to the starting point.

SEMO Drill

The SEMO drill is another good functional test that involves all of the previously mentioned movement patterns (Kirby, 1971; see Figure 3.16). This drill is usually performed within the free throw lane of a basketball court, but any other similar area may be used. Set markers in each of the four corners of the free throw lane. Facing away from the free throw line, starting at marker A, the athlete side-shuffles right to marker B. Pivoting off the left foot at marker B, the athlete backpedals diagonally across the free throw lane to marker C. Planting and accelerating

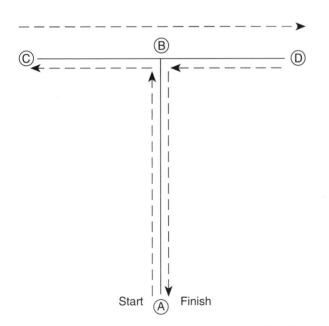

Figure 3.15 The T-shuffle or T-cut can be performed for uniform testing distances or sport-specific distances.

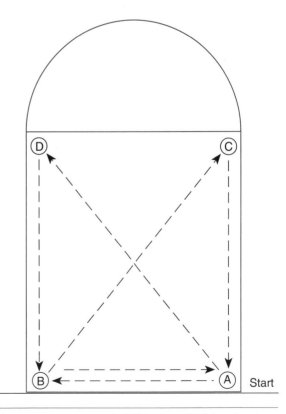

Figure 3.16 The SEMO drill is a practical functional test incorporating forward, backward, and diagonal acceleration along with lateral movement.

off the right foot, he or she then sprints forward to marker A. At marker A, the athlete plants and accelerates off the right foot and backpedals across the lane to marker D. At marker D, he or she sprints forward to marker B, then side-shuffles left to starting point A. This is a fantastic drill for athletes required to change directions quickly.

Co-Contraction Test

The co-contraction test, a special test to dynamically assess functional stability of the unstable knee, has been recently developed (Lephart, Perrin, Fu, & Minger, 1991). This test and its modifications are valuable in testing the anterior cruciate deficient athlete. Using heavy rubber tubing anchored to a secure base and attached to the athlete, resistance is applied as the athlete backs up, placing more tension in the rubber tube. Maintaining this posterior directed force, the athlete side-steps or shuffles around an 8-foot radius about the fixed rubber tube (see Figure 3.17).

A modification of this test uses not only the posterior force created against the forward pull of the tubing but also forward and backward acceleration and deceleration and the lateral shuffling component of the co-contraction test.

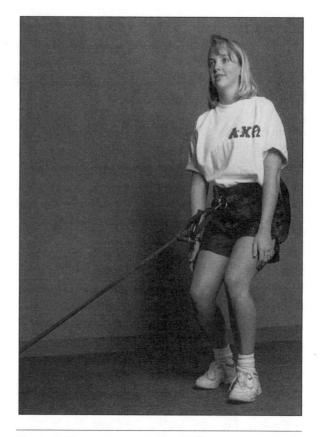

Figure 3.17   Surgical tubing is anchored to a stable object and then secured around the athlete's waist. Exerting posterior force against the tube requires co-contraction of the muscles around the knee to provide dynamic joint stability.

♦ Summary

Functional testing, like functional progression, is limited only by your imagination. You must always have the demands of the specific sport in mind. A standardized method of measurement is important, as well as a keen eye for substitution.

The vital prerequisites for specific functional progressions have been provided. You now know the general principles of functional progression as well as the scientific foundations on which they are based. This understanding will serve as a framework in building a sport readiness program. Although movement patterns and skills, physical demands, participation time restraints, and other concerns all differ from sport to sport, you can apply general functional progression principles to all sporting activities. With these basics behind us, let's move to the sport-specific functional progression programs for collision and contact, combat, jumping, throwing, and running sports.

PART II

Functional Progression for Specific Sports

$\blacklozenge\blacklozenge$

Part I laid the groundwork from which to build a functional progression program. Program basics, the neurophysiology of closed-chain functional exercise, and functional testing were discussed. Now it is time to add to these fundamental principles and apply them as you plan functional programs for specific sports.

The specific activities we'll look at are divided into collision and contact sports, jumping sports, combat sports, throwing sports, and running sports. These categories include the majority of activities you will be exposed to in the sport rehabilitation program. Guidelines to follow will serve as the framework for you to construct your own functional progression programs. Keep in mind that the following chapters are guidelines only—do not feel tied to these programs. Every athlete and every injury is unique; rehabilitation should be unique also. Get a good feel for the principles involved and modify the programs to fit your needs. Adapting the program to each patient will help ensure a consummate return to function.

CHAPTER 4

♦♦♦

Collision and Contact Sports

Many sports involve body contact and now and then an inadvertent collision. However, with the sports discussed in this chapter body contact is forceful and necessary to the game. Before we proceed, an explanation of the differences between collision sports and contact sports might be helpful.

♦ Collision Sports

Collision sports are those that promote physical contact between players. This contact is usually one player's deliberate attempt to impede another player's progress. Usually, collision sports are team sports in which one team attempts to control the opposing team's territory. Physical contact is necessary as players try to gain ground in the opposing team's territory and prevent their own territory from being taken by the opponent. When the opponent's territory has been taken, points are usually awarded. For example, the goal of an American football team is to stay within the confines of the playing field and cross the opposing team's goal line for a touchdown, worth 6 points. In hockey, six players face off against each other to try to put the hockey puck into the goal of the opposing team, which scores 1 point.

Collision sports enjoying popularity are American football, hockey, lacrosse, and rugby. Collision sports combine speed, strength, and agility with power and anaerobic and aerobic fitness. The result is a fast-paced, high-impact sport in which injury is a strong possibility. Sophisticated protective equipment dramatically decreases certain types of injury in collision sports. However, macrotraumatic injury is still common in collision sports. Partial or complete ligament sprains and muscle strains occur frequently. Bone fractures and dislocations and subluxations of joints also happen fairly often. A list of common joints injured, along with the mechanism of specific injuries, can be found in Table 4.1.

♦ Contact Sports

Contact sports contain occasional forceful physical bumping between opposing players, but this contact is uncommon and is usually against the rules of the game. Many contact sports are also territorial, but physical contact is not the primary means of protecting one's territory or gaining ground in the opponent's territory. Contact sports enjoying worldwide popularity include soccer and team handball. Other popular contact sports are basketball, baseball, softball, and wrestling. These sports and others will be discussed in following chapters dealing with jumping, throwing, and combat sports, respectively.

♦ Rehabilitation Concerns

The acute management of macrotrauma, though vital to the overall success of a rehab program, is not within the scope of this book. If you are responsible for the acute management of sport injury, you must be able to implement appropriate evaluation and care. If you are not primarily responsible for the immediate management, you will see the athlete when it is time to institute the rehabilitation program. Rehabilitation concerns key to successful and comprehensive athletic rehabilitation after injury sustained in a collision or contact sport should be mentioned here. Table 4.2 contains a list of injuries common to collision and contact sports, along with prime concerns for your rehabilitation program prior to instituting functional progression. Once you are ready to begin functional progression efforts, the remainder of the chapter will be of significant benefit.

Table 4.1   Common Injuries in Contact and Collision Sports

Body area	Injury	Mechanism of injury
Acromioclavicular joint	Sprain	Fall onto point of shoulder
	"Separated shoulder"	Fall on hand of outstretched arm
Glenohumeral joint	Sprain	Fall on hand of outstretched arm
		Forceful horizontal abduction to externally rotated/abducted arm
Brachialis muscle belly	Contusion	Direct trauma
Iliac crest	Contusion ("hip pointer")	Direct trauma, fall
Quadriceps muscle belly	Contusion	Direct trauma
Knee joint		
Tibial collateral ligament	Sprain	Valgus stress
Distal femoral epiphysis	Fracture	Valgus stress
Anterior cruciate ligament	Sprain	Valgus/varus stress with rotation
		Hyperextension, hyperflexion
Meniscus	Tear	Rotation of weight-bearing leg
		Hyperextension, hyperflexion
Ankle joint	Sprain	Inversion/eversion with plantar or dorsi flexion
Metatarsalphalangeal joint	Sprain ("turf-toe")	Hyperextension

Table 4.2   Rehabilitation Concerns for Contact/Collision Sport Injuries

Injury	Rehabilitation concerns
Acromioclavicular sprain	Anterior deltoid strengthening; protective padding
Glenohumeral subluxation/dislocation	Humeral positioner strengthening and proprioception activities
Brachialis contusion	Judicious use of heat and stretching; customized protective padding
Iliac crest contusion	Gluteus medius and oblique abdominal stretching; protective padding
Quadriceps contusion	Judicious use of heat and stretching; customized protective padding
Tibial collateral ligament sprain	Aggressive quadriceps strengthening, graduated valgus loading
Anterior cruciate ligament sprain	Protected quadriceps strengthening; supranormal hamstring strengthening, functional knee bracing; proprioception activities
Meniscus tear	Protected quadriceps strengthening; proprioception activities
Inversion ankle sprain	Aggressive evertor and dorsiflexor strengthening; calf stretching; taping/bracing; proprioception activities

♦ Lower Extremity

What follows are functional progression guidelines for the athlete with a lower extremity injury. Table 4.3 contains a helpful checklist to assist you in progressing your athletes following lower extremity injury. Each step in Table 4.3 is a given skill (or set of skills) unique to itself. The athlete must progress through each group of skills before advancing to the next skill or group of skills. For example, the athlete must first conquer bilateral support skills before moving to unilateral support skills. Particular skills to consider within each of the steps in Table 4.3 are found in the text. As discussed in chapter 1, skills are only progressed as the athlete tolerates.

Unloaded Activities

As mentioned in chapter 1, in unloaded activities the athlete receives no added resistance in the performance of a specific skill. Although in contact and collision sports an opponent might be banging off of the individual, preliminary activities that do not

Table 4.3   Functional Progression Checklist for Lower Extremity Injury

Unloaded activities	Loaded activities
_____ Graduated weight-bearing activities and conditioning	_____ Bilateral support drills
_____ Bilateral support drills	_____ Unilateral support drills
_____ Unilateral support drills	_____ Bilateral nonsupport drills
_____ Bilateral nonsupport drills	_____ Unilateral nonsupport drills
_____ Unilateral nonsupport drills	_____ Single-plane one-on-one force delivery and force acceptance drills
_____ Running/sprinting program	_____ Multiplane one-on-one force delivery and force acceptance drills
_____ Acceleration/deceleration pivoting drills	_____ Single-plane two-on-one force delivery and force acceptance drills
	_____ Multiplane two-on-one force delivery and force acceptance drills
	_____ Group force acceptance drills

stress physical contact must be included in the program as well. The majority of action in collision and contact sports involve loaded activities, but it is important to establish a strong fundamental base of unloaded activities that must be met by all players, especially those in "skilled" positions who play key roles on the team. It is crucial to the team's success that the players in skilled positions possess the highest possible degree of speed and agility. Examples of skilled positions are the quarterback and the offensive and defensive backfield players in American football, and the forwards and goalkeepers in soccer, hockey, and lacrosse.

Support Drills

During the unloaded portion of functional progression emphasize smooth, reciprocating, weight-bearing activities. Once athletes can perform bilateral and unilateral support drills, aggressive retraining in the specific footwork required for their position should be drilled over and over again. These activities are performed at speeds at least 50% of normal speed. Your focus is on a smooth transition of weight bearing from the noninvolved lower extremity to the involved side. Full-speed footwork drills will not be allowed until the athlete has progressed through the acceleration/deceleration pivoting sequence. Initially these activities should take place with no other players in proximity and with no equipment. For example, the athlete should do simple footwork drills in isolation

without a football, soccer ball, or hockey stick. Only after they have successfully completed the basic footwork skills should athletes begin drills with another player or equipment.

For all athletes in collision and contact sports, cardiovascular and musculoskeletal endurance should be emphasized early in the unloaded segment of functional progression. Unfortunately, this area is often ignored. As soon as the individual can bear weight on the affected leg, pool running, cycling, and other means to stress the cardiovascular and musculoskeletal endurance systems should begin. For specifics, refer to Table 7.3 on page 85.

A related basic concept also frequently overlooked is addressing the appropriate energy system when working on cardiovascular and musculoskeletal endurance. It is essential to have the athlete try to maintain aerobic endurance with workouts at 60% to 85% of maximum predicted heart rate for 20 to 30 minutes. However, you must remember that most collision and contact sports are primarily anaerobic in nature. If you stress only the aerobic energy system during the rehabilitation program, you have short-changed the athlete.

Make sport-specific anaerobic bursts of energy a part of your rehabilitation program. If football line play is under 10 seconds, or a routine hockey shift from 30 to 45 seconds, stress repetitive conditioning drills accordingly. Soccer and lacrosse players are typically on the playing field longer, but they are required to expend quick bursts of energy as well.

The drills you include in functional progression programs for these athletes should also have sport-specific energy requirements.

Nonsupport Drills

Keeping both feet on the ground at almost all times is necessary in most collision and contact sports. With one foot off the ground, the athlete's base of support is greatly decreased and the chance of being upended increased. However, unilateral weight bearing while remaining balanced enough to adequately function is a requirement for athletes playing both skilled and nonskilled positions. The football defensive lineman's ability to jump when trying to block a pass is important, as is the soccer defender attempting to head a ball away from the front of the goal. Therefore, bilateral and then unilateral nonsupport drills should be included in functional progression for athletes of all collision and contact sports.

As with support drills, athletes beginning nonsupport drills should be isolated from teammates and use no equipment. Equipment can be introduced later to make the drills more functional. For example, the injured soccer player can progress from simple front-to-back and side-to-side jumping and hopping done in isolation, to performing the same drills while heading the ball back to a teammate. Once stationary front-to-back and side-to-side drills are no longer difficult for the athlete, add additional stress by having him or her perform higher jumps or hops over a ball (see Figure 4.1).

Acceleration/Deceleration/Pivoting Sequence

During this phase it is not difficult to make each drill sport and position specific. Sport distances, directions, and speeds can be easily duplicated to suit the athlete you are working with. If the athlete must perform in a relatively small area (e.g., football interior linemen or lacrosse and soccer goal keepers), the distances for acceleration and deceleration maneuvers should be kept small. On the other hand, if distances are greater, (e.g., football offensive and defensive backs and pass receivers), acceleration and deceleration activities should be performed over greater distances. Straight ahead, backward, and lateral movements should be performed in a single plane, and progressed to combinations of movements.

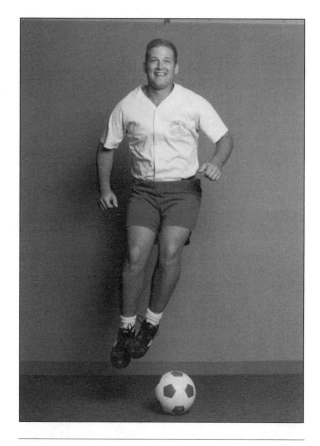

Figure 4.1 Front-to-back, side-to-side, and diagonal line jumping and hopping can be integrated with sport equipment or sport drills.

An excellent activity during this phase is the *mirror drill.* In this drill, the athlete performs the identical movement of another player or a coach, or a therapist. When possible, you should put the individual through the drill yourself to assess performance firsthand. Movements to stress in mirror drills are quick changes of direction from front-to-back and side-to-side and forward and backward diagonals. You can perform the desired movement and have the athlete mimic you, or you can indicate the desired movement with hand signals. Again, these movements should be sport specific and performed over a distance that the athlete will be required to cover upon return to sport. Simple pivoting and cutting drills (see pages 15-18 in chapter 1) should be the bare minimum required before proceeding to loaded activities. You are encouraged to go one step further with sport-specific functional drills. Football offensive receivers should be able to run normal pass patterns. Hockey, lacrosse, and soccer players should be able to perform every basic movement pattern required of their position before proceeding to loaded activities.

Once the athlete has mastered these activities, one more transitional step should be put into play prior to starting loaded activities. Before the athlete resumes contact drills, he or she should perform unloaded activities with all required protective equipment in place. The equipment places extra weight on the injured body part and readies the athlete for resuming loaded activities.

Loaded Activities

The basic functional progression program in chapter 1 concluded with the athlete satisfactorily performing acceleration/deceleration and pivoting maneuvers. What happens to the rugby player who must deliver and absorb physical contact as part of the sport? Athletes in collision and contact sports must be ready for the physical contact inherent in their sport. The unloaded segment of functional progression ensures that all movement patterns required of the athlete are performed normally. Now you must ready the individual for physical contact.

It is essential that these next steps in the loaded section of functional progression are properly advanced. When the collision or contact athlete reaches the point to once again put the body on the line, you need to be aware of two potentially abnormal psychological reactions the athlete may exhibit. At one end of the spectrum, an athlete may seem totally oblivious to the resolving injury, wanting to get back to full activity, throwing all caution to the wind. On the other end of the spectrum, you may work with athletes who worry too much about reinjury. The desired state of mind lies somewhere between the two. You want the athlete aggressive and performing at preinjury level without worrying about the current injury, but you do not want the athlete to repeat the kind of mistake that caused the injury (if in fact there was a mistake). For athletes who are tentative, you want them to understand that all that can be done to prepare for their return to activity has been done. These athletes need to overcome tentativeness to be effective.

So the transition from unloaded to loaded activities is not to be taken lightly. Do not get caught up in the glamour of returning an athlete to sport early just because the athlete is moving well and is well-motivated. Channel the motivation properly toward the safe completion of the loaded segment of the functional progression program. On the other hand, do not become overly concerned and feed an athlete's excess worry. Reassure the athlete that a safe return to sport is just as close as completing the loaded functional progression program.

Certain sport-related equipment can assist a smooth transition to contact drills. Football blocking sleds, stationary blocking and tackling dummies, as well as hand-held dummies may all be used to stress contact and collision with a decreased force component. The heavy stationary dummies are held resting on the ground and serve as a nonmoving target for the recuperating athlete to block or tackle. The lighter hand-held dummies can be held by the injured athlete to serve as a buffer. This equipment can also be utilized in the functional progression program for other sports.

Simply put, during the loaded phase of functional progression, the athlete must be able both to provide and to accept force. In this phase, the athlete must be able to generate sufficient force for sport performance and also withstand forces of competition magnitude.

Collision sports often involve activities in which one athlete is pitted against more than one opponent. The scrum in rugby, a gang tackle in football, or a pile-up in front of the hockey net all involve multiple participants. You must make multiple participant activities part of the loaded functional progression program. Loaded activities should begin one on one, with the recuperating athlete matched against a single opponent. Once one-on-one drills have been mastered, you may progress the athlete to two-on-one situations, and finally to group contact activities. Let's look at specific ways to progress your athletes through a loaded functional progression program after a lower extremity injury.

To make physical contact effective in collision and contact sports, the athlete's ability to deliver force must be maximized. A strong blocker or tackler is usually more effective and at less risk for injury than a weaker blocker or tackler. The same holds true when an athlete must accept contact. An individual with strength to absorb the force is less likely to be injured and is usually more effective than a weaker opponent. Therefore, early efforts in the loaded functional progression should emphasize force delivery and force acceptance.

Force delivery can be defined as an individual imparting force to an opponent. In American football, force delivery involves blocking, tackling, and other forms of forceful contact. Rugby and lacrosse involve similar types of activities. Hockey allows for "checking," the term for contact with the opponent. Colliding with opponents to impede their progress is frowned on in soccer. However, contact is allowed when the soccer player "tackles" the opponent in an attempt to take the ball away. *Force acceptance* involves being tackled, blocked, or checked, or receiving another kind of a blow from an opponent.

Single-Plane Force Delivery and Acceptance

Force delivery and acceptance should begin in a controlled environment. Just as in unloaded activities, the parameters of speed and movement must be advanced with common sense. Speeds should initially be kept low, and movement must start in single planes. The added component of force delivery and acceptance should also be advanced using common sense. That is, low forces at slow speeds in single-plane movements should progress to greater forces at faster speeds in multiple planes of movement.

• **Speed.** As with unloaded acceleration and deceleration skills, speeds should be advanced from a jogging pace, to half-speed sprinting, and finally to full-speed activities. Speeds should be kept slow, initially walking through blocking, tackling, or checking drills. Once lower extremity movement patterns are appropriate as the individual makes contact at walking speeds, the speed of the drill can be increased.

• **Distance.** Distances should be specific to position. For example, the football lineman should concentrate on distances appropriate for line play (3 to 5 yards) and advance to downfield blocking. Football offensive and defensive backfield players and pass receivers should work on distances of 8 to 12 yards and advance to downfield tackling and being tackled drills. Hockey players should work the entire length of the ice. Soccer, lacrosse, and team handball players should all be able to cover the entire length of the playing field. Distances prior to force delivery and force acceptance should be no greater than 1 yard. Of special concern during this phase is a stable base of support. You must stress to

the athlete the importance of a substantial base of support. Feet should be slightly greater than shoulder-width apart, hips and knees should be flexed slightly, and body weight should be centered over the balls of the feet.

• **Duration.** Drill duration should approximate normal playing time. If a maximal series of play involves 12 to 15 plays, then 12 to 15 repetitions of the drill should be performed. Likewise, if the typical playing time is 45 seconds, allow for 45 seconds of functional progression activities. It is also important to allow for a typical recovery time between drills. If the sport involves 10 to 15 seconds of maximal activity followed by 45 seconds of rest, make sure the functional progression follows suit.

• **Pairing.** Match participants for height and weight. Efforts should be one on one, with the recuperating individual paired with a teammate of similar height and weight. In this consideration, weight is certainly more important than height. To minimize chances of reinjury, match a 200-pound athlete with another 200-pounder. Try to keep in mind the athlete's height also, as a mismatch certainly occurs in the case of a 6'5" 200-pounder against a 5'9" 200-pounder.

• **Single Plane.** Keep force delivery and acceptance in a single plane. Drills should initially be stressed in a single plane. This means that the two individuals should perform blocking, tackling, and checking drills straight on, one participant directly in front of the other. Drills can then be progressed to being performed directly from the side. Single-plane movements allow the athlete direct visual awareness of the teammate.

Multiplane Force Delivery and Acceptance

In the one-on-one section of loaded drills, the final progression should be performed in multiple planes. In the previous drills, movement has been kept in a single plane to allow the individual to prepare for the force delivery or acceptance. Now the individual should be prepared for multiplane drills, which will not only add different stresses to the healing tissue, but also add an element of surprise. You are now asking the athlete to react to the unexpected. Checking, blocking, and tackling drills will be performed at angles that decrease the involved athlete's visual awareness of the opponent.

When appropriate, drills can then be progressed from behind, where the athlete is less able to prepare for the physical contact.

Because many activities in collision and contact sports involve more than one-on-one encounters, you must ready the sport participant for two-on-one activities. Program guidelines are the same as previously discussed in the one-on-one section, but this time an additional athlete is added to the drills. The individual should be able to deliver force with the assistance of a teammate and to accept force from two opposing players. Don't forget to

• Match the athletes for height and weight.

• Emphasize sport-specific function.

• Keep initial distances short (less than 1 yard) and progress to greater distances as dictated by the athlete's position.

• Progress speeds from jogging, to a half-speed sprint, and finally to full speed.

• Expose the athlete to game-type experience. The best test is practice or scrimmage sessions. At this time a good rapport with the coaching or athletic training staff is vital. With the assistance of these essential personnel, the athlete can be exposed to game-type situations in a controlled environment. Normal position requirements that stress coordinated team timing is the final test before returning the athlete to competition. Careful observation with the help of a nonbiased, trained observer is essential at this stage.

♦ Upper Extremity

As with the functional progression program following lower extremity injury, upper extremity functional progression can also be divided into loaded and unloaded drills. It is easy to picture lower extremity loaded and unloaded activities. But it is a little more difficult to envision loaded upper extremity function. Before proceeding, let's discuss loaded versus unloaded activities as they relate to upper extremity function.

Unloaded Activities

In the first chapter, you learned that unloaded activities pertain to those skills in which no outside resistance is applied to the individual. Loaded activities, on the other hand, involve those skills where the athlete takes on added resistance in the form of heavy equipment or another player. When discussing functional progression activities after lower extremity injury, the difference between loaded and unloaded skills is obvious. The picture becomes blurry when discussing upper extremity loaded and unloaded drills. Traditionally, the upper extremity is not thought of as a weight-bearing joint. However, to stimulate certain mechanoreceptors and facilitate proprioception, weight bearing is a must. Therefore, you must think in terms of upper extremity weight bearing as the starting point of functional progression. These unloaded activities must be stressed before giving way to loaded activities. Loaded upper extremity drills are those in which weight plus outside resistance is accepted on the involved arm. Let's look at some specifics of upper extremity functional progressions for the contact and collision athlete. Once again, do not let these guidelines stifle your thinking. Be innovative and add to the basics that follow.

Bilateral Support Drills

Basic concepts of the functional progression do not change. After injury to the upper extremity, weight-bearing activities begin on both arms. Upper extremity weight-bearing skills can be more difficult to observe for symmetry, substitution, and balance. Keen observation skills are vital to ensure that athletes are performing the desired task correctly. It is sometimes necessary to observe them while straddling them. Other times you will need to get down on the floor with an athlete as he or she performs. Bilateral support drills simply involve weight shift of the body over the fixed upper extremities in a modified 4-point (hands and knees) position. Initial activities should be with the elbows extended to allow for additional stabilization through the shoulder girdle and trunk (see Figure 4.2a). Once the athlete can demonstrate symmetrical weight acceptance through both arms in a front-to-back and side-to-side rocking fashion through a limited range, additional range of motion can be added. Elbow flexion may now be allowed to facilitate a greater arc of motion and decrease the stability afforded by the trunk (see Figure 4.2b). This modified push-up

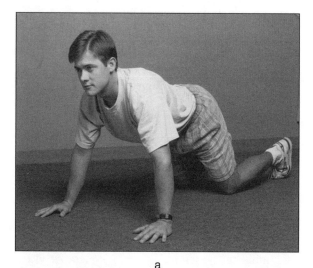

a

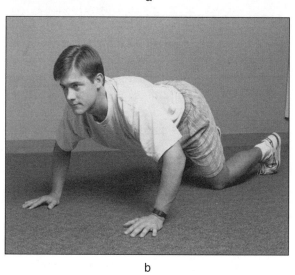

b

Figure 4.2 (a) Elbow extension to impart loading through the shoulder girdle. (b) Flexed elbows allow greater stress through the elbows.

position is a natural extension of early weight-bearing activity and beneficial as a core stability position for bilateral weight acceptance.

Stability in the 4-point position is mandatory before moving on. A stable 4-point base is a prerequisite before progressing to forward, backward, or lateral movements in the 4-point stance. A great way to encourage additional weight bearing with movement on both upper extremities is the up-and-down drill.

Up-and-Down Drill

To perform the up-and-down drill, the athlete alternates from a standing position on both feet, to a

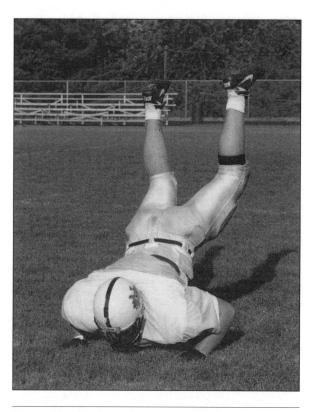

Figure 4.3 The up-and-down drill increases force on the upper extremities through weight acceptance in the down position and ground reaction force pushing back up into the standing position.

push-up position, and then back onto the feet again (see Figure 4.3). Up-and-down drills add momentum to weight-bearing forces through the arms and also place an eccentric muscle load as the shoulder girdle musculature decelerates the body safely to the push-up position.

Up-and-down drills can be made more difficult by having the athlete jog forward to a set spot and then perform the drill. A distance of 3 to 5 yards is used. The athlete jogs the distance, performs an up-and-down, jogs another 3 to 5 yards, does another up-and-down, and repeats the sequence a designated total distance or for a sport-specific duration. As with lower extremity progression, speeds can be increased to half-sprint, and then to full sprinting.

Crawling Drill

Crawling activities on hands and knees are also excellent ways to encourage weight bearing through the involved arm and stress a transition to unilateral weight bearing and reciprocating motion. Initially, crawling should be done on hands and knees, and

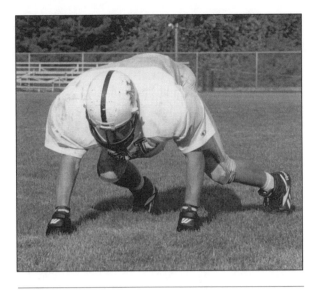

Figure 4.4 Bear-crawling increases force through the upper extremities without lower extremity support. This crawl also causes repetitive cyclic loading and unloading of the arms.

then advanced to hands and feet (bear) crawling (see Figure 4.4).

Remember to keep within functional progression guidelines. Activities should first be performed in a single direction, either front to back or side to side. Crawling should also be progressed from half speed to three-fourths speed to full speed. Although useful as a functional progression tool, crawling is not specific to many sports, so it is difficult to have the athlete crawl for sport-specific distances. Rather, the athlete should crawl for sport-specific periods of time. Have the athlete perform for the average length of time that a play will last and for the average number of plays required of a specific position. Be sure to provide adequate recovery time.

Wheelbarrow Drill

Another modification of crawling is the wheelbarrow position. Have a teammate lift the patient's legs off of the ground and hold onto them as the patient steps with his or her arms (see Figure 4.5). This activity may seem borderline childish, but it requires the individual to support virtually entire body weight on the arms and simultaneously absorb reciprocating forces directed up the injured arm. Once again, these activities may be performed front to back, side to side, and then in multiplane directions. Progressions regarding distance and duration are the same as described for crawling activities.

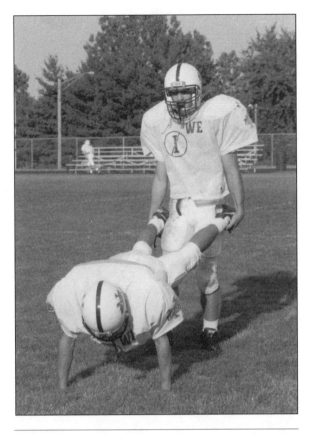

Figure 4.5 Additional force is imparted through the upper extremities through the added vertical component afforded by the partner providing control of the legs.

Inverted Push-Up

Perhaps the most aggressive bilateral support upper extremity drill is a modification of the inverted push-up. Since essentially all of the athlete's weight is placed through the arms, great upper body strength is required to perform this activity correctly. This skill may be too aggressive for the functional progression program but, modified, can be a stimulating way to strengthen the athlete for unilateral weight-bearing activity. Graduated positions as shown in Figure 4.6 can be used to develop the strength to perform this drill. In cases where sport-specific periods of time are excessive for this drill, sets and repetitions may be substituted.

Please keep in mind the injured tissue when having athletes perform these drills. Yes, you want to stress the injured tissue to facilitate optimum healing, but never place the athlete at risk for jeopardizing the status of the injured tissue. Refer to Table 4.4 for specific positions to avoid after common upper extremity injuries.

Table 4.4 Upper Extremity Positional Precautions

Upper extremity condition	Position/activity precaution
Posterior shoulder instability	Heavy bench press (unrack position) Finish position of push-ups, hands and knees position with elbows locked
Anterior shoulder instability	Heavy bench press (bar at chest position) Extremes of horizontal abduction (especially heavy loaded)
Inferior shoulder instability	Heavy overhead activity (military press) Inverted push-ups
Acromioclavicular instability	Force delivery/acceptance on tip of shoulder
Sternoclavicular instability	Extremes of horizontal adduction or abduction (especially heavy loaded)

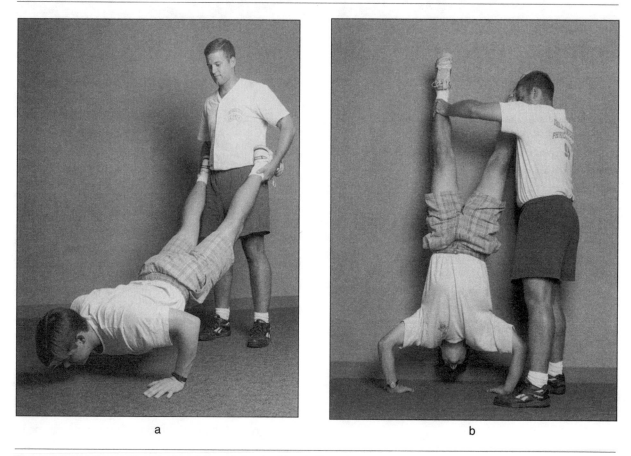

a   b

Figure 4.6   (a) Greater force is placed through the shoulder girdle as the athlete is supported with the trunk parallel to the floor. (b) Tremendous strength is required for the inverted push-up. Remember precautions for the individual with shoulder instability.

Transitional Drills

Sometimes an athlete may progress beyond bilateral support drills but not yet be ready for unilateral support efforts. In such cases, try bilateral efforts with less support from the noninvolved side and with controlled added momentum. Two examples of these efforts are in using the Shuttle 2001 or in doing wall rebounding drills. In each of these, momentum provides added resistance to the athlete

in an easily controlled environment. Both seated efforts on the Shuttle (see Figure 4.7a) and standing wall rebounds (see Figure 4.7b) can be performed for sport-specific lengths of time.

Unilateral Support Drills

Similar to lower extremity functional progression, unilateral support drills are simple modifications of bilateral support activities. Single-arm work should

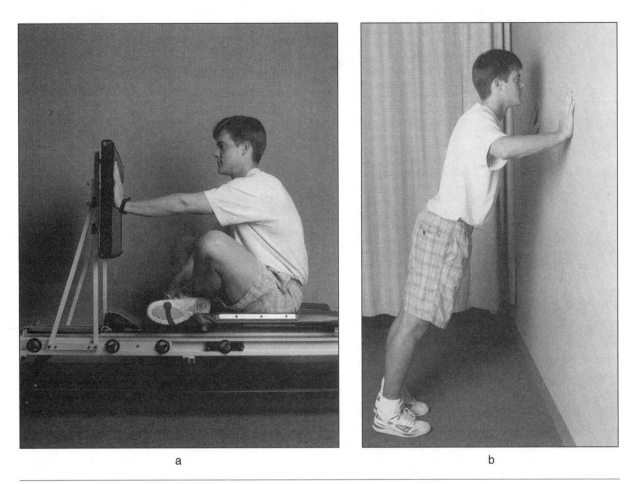

a   b

Figure 4.7 (a) Unilateral support drill on the Shuttle 2001. (b) Bilateral nonsupport drill with standing wall rebounds.

begin in a stationary 3-point position as shown in Figure 4.8.

Initial skills should emphasize front-to-back and side-to-side rocking motions. The involved arm should, of course, be the weight-bearing arm. Beginning skills should be with the elbow extended. As strength and weight acceptance improves, a slight amount of elbow flexion can be added as the individual is asked to shift body weight over a larger area. Unilateral push-ups can be added with the individual beginning on one arm and both knees and progressing to the traditional push-up position.

Arm Hopping and Spins

Unilateral wheelbarrow drills are not practical, but there is a good way to facilitate unilateral weight bearing with superimposed body movement. Two such drills are arm hopping and arm spins.

Arm hopping is a modification of the up-and-down drill for distance (see page 54). This time

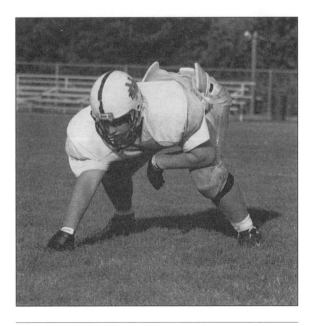

Figure 4.8 Single-arm support places added stress through the shoulder girdle. Watch for substitutions from excessive trunk flexion.

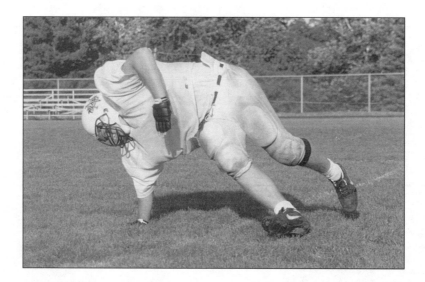

Figure 4.9   This unilateral support drill for the upper extremity places added stress compared to the single-arm support, as the athlete "walks" in clockwise and counterclockwise circles through the weight-bearing arm.

instead of jogging to a spot and performing the up-and-down on both arms, the athlete supports the body weight on both legs and the involved arm only. The athlete jogs to the set spot, accepts full weight on the involved arm, allows the elbow to flex slightly, pushes off the arm, and jogs to the next spot. Speeds and distances can be increased as the athlete tolerates.

Arm spins are stationary drills in which the athlete assumes full weight on the involved arm, with elbow extended and lower body weight supported on the balls of the feet (see Figure 4.9). While maintaining this position, the athlete spins clockwise and counterclockwise around the fixed arm. Quick changes of direction are encouraged as the athlete performs the drill for a sport-specific length of time.

Forward Rolls

Being able to gradually accept weight on the tip of the shoulder is especially beneficial for collision and contact athletes who have sustained acro-mioclavicular injury. Gentle forward rolls are excellent for stressing the shoulder in this way. As with all functional progression drills, moderation and a gradual increase in intensity is the rule. Forward rolls should be stressed first from a hands and knees position. The athlete kneels on both knees using the opposite hand for support, tucks the involved shoulder, and places the shoulder tip on the floor (see Figure 4.10). From this position, the athlete performs a forward roll. Natural progression for this activity is initiating the roll from a squatting position, and then to a standing position. Once the forward roll is mastered from a standing position, the athlete can jog and then perform the roll. Multiple forward rolls in succession can be performed over a given distance. As proficiency improves, increase speed.

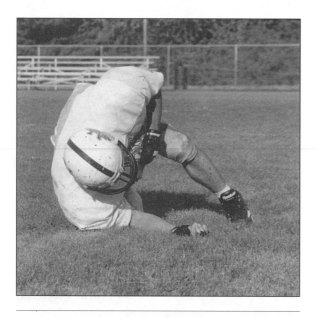

Figure 4.10   Beginning in the quadruped position, the athlete accepts weight on the involved shoulder and then rolls the body over the fixed shoulder girdle complex. Forces can be added by progressing to the stationary standing position and then to a moving upright position.

Loaded Activities

Now that the athlete has progressed through the unloaded sequence of upper extremity functional progression, you can add extraneous resistance. In collision and contact sports, athletes must be able to supply force and to absorb force through the arm. Grabbing, pushing, pulling, shoving, and tackling are but some of the necessary functions in contact and collision sports. You can readily employ sport-specific functions to prepare the individual for upper extremity demands.

Blocking sleds, stationary blocking dummies, heavy punching bags, or medicine balls can all be employed to reproduce force acceptance and force delivery skills. Adequate lower extremity base of support, with the hips and knees slightly flexed and body weight over the balls of the feet, will aid in maximizing upper extremity force delivery and force acceptance. Stationary objects should be used to allow the injured athlete to deliver force. The athlete may approach the stationary blocking sled or tackling dummy and deliver submaximal to maximal forces through bilateral upper extremities. Moving objects can be used to assist the athlete in accepting force. The medicine ball can be thrown at the athlete, or the heavy punching bag may be swung at him or her. After force acceptance, the athlete can then deliver force by throwing the ball or pushing the bag. As with other functional progression drills, distances can be increased as well as the speed in which force is accepted or delivered.

One-On-One Drills

Sport-specific drills stressing upper extremity force acceptance and delivery can effectively be done with teammates. The activities should begin with the individual working with a teammate of approximately the same height and weight. Drills should begin at walking speeds and should be stressed in a single plane.

Straight-On Drills

Straight-on drills should be done with a teammate walking toward the recuperating individual. The injured athlete should accept the contact from the teammate with bilateral upper extremities, allow minimal elbow flexion, and then deliver sufficient force to push the teammate away (see Figure 4.11).

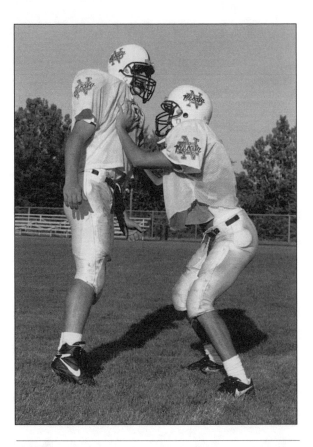

Figure 4.11 Force acceptance through the shoulder girdle should emphasize the ready position of wrist extension, elbow flexion, and scapular protraction.

Emphasize adequate lower leg support and a coordinated, symmetrical response from the upper extremities (see Figure 4.12).

Keeping with functional progression guidelines, the speed with which the teammate approaches should be increased gradually to full speed. Distances covered should be sport-specific. Football offensive and defensive linemen may work in distances of 3 to 5 yards. Hockey players, on the other hand, may need to work over larger distances on the ice to approximate normal playing forces.

Multiple Teammate Drill

Another helpful drill in readying athletes of collision and contact sports for competition is doing straight-ons with multiple teammates. Force is applied by only one teammate at a time, but different teammates take turns approaching the injured athlete from different angles. During this drill, the athlete should be fully aware which teammate is approaching to apply force. But emphasis is placed on reacting to the various angles while accepting and delivering force through the upper extremities. In this drill, the athlete stands with at least three other players encircling her or him. The athlete

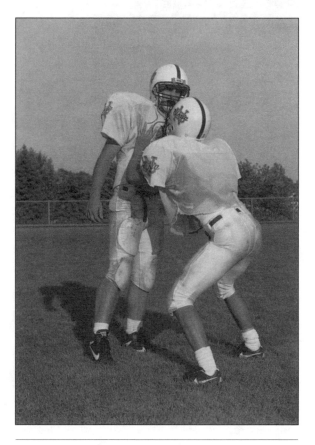

Figure 4.12   To adequately dissipate the force to be accepted a stable base of support is a must.

assumes a stable base of support, and the teammates each approach one at a time in a set sequence (see Figure 4.13). Once again, as proficiency improves, speed and distance are increased to increase force. This is a great drill performed on either land or ice.

Up to now emphasis has been placed on single, controlled force delivery and acceptance. But upper extremity function in collision and contact sports is not always isolated. Players of hockey, football, team handball, and rugby must also be able to grab, pull, and tackle. Still using one-on-one drills, now stress these activities. Tackling and grasping drills should be performed with the same progression guidelines in mind. These activities are stressed by emphasizing proper form. The injured athlete's initial contact is made on a stationary teammate; the hands are then used in sport-specific fashion to secure the teammate. As discussed previously, distances should be sport-specific, participants should be matched to size, and initial activities should be straight-on or from the side. Speed and distance is increased gradually to maximum speeds and distances encountered in competition. To add a degree of unexpectedness, after these skills have been mastered, progress to grabbing, tackling, and pulling drills performed in multiplane directions.

Two-on-One Drills

After satisfactorily progressing through multiplane one-on-one force delivery and acceptance drills, you must now ready the athlete for group collision and contact. Gang tackles in football, the rugby

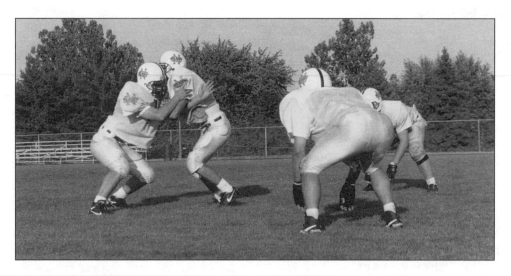

Figure 4.13   This reaction drill emphasizes multiplane force acceptance as the athlete must accept force from three individuals coming from varying directions at different times.

scrum, or a group of hockey players clenched around a puck "frozen" against the boards all involve more than one body exerting force against the individual. Although some of these situations are not readily reproducible until scrimmage sessions, you can stress them in controlled two-on-one functional progression activities. These activities are similar to those found in the one-on-one section. The athlete must be able to absorb force from and deliver force to two teammates. Such activities can easily be performed in double-team blocking and tackling drills in football, or checking drills in hockey. Remember that the recuperating athlete must be able both to assist in the blocking and tackling with a teammate and to be blocked and tackled by two teammates. As always, speeds are started slow and gradually progressed. Distance should be kept sport-specific, and efforts should begin in a single plane and progress to multiplane efforts. Finally, after conquering two-on-one activities, the athlete is ready for controlled scrimmages, in which situations resemble real competition.

◆ Special Considerations

Most common collision and contact sports have "specialty" players, of which there are two kinds. One kind of specialty player plays a team position that does not resemble the other positions. Examples are kickers and punters in American football and goal keepers in hockey, soccer, team handball, and lacrosse. (The quarterback in American football is also a specialty player; functional progression for a return to throwing can be found in chapter 8.)

The other kind of specialty player is one involved on a special team in a given sport. Examples are members of the kickoff team, kick-receiving team, or extra-point team in American football and the penalty-killing team and power-play team in hockey.

Specialty players have unique demands placed on them, so their functional progression program must be specialized as well. All specialty players must be able to pass through the unloaded program following lower extremity injury.

Kicking and Foot Skills

Unloaded activities stress unilateral weight acceptance drills and proceed to acceleration and decel-

eration activities. Kicking athletes, whether they are specialty players in football (kicker or punter) or position players in soccer or rugby who are required to kick as well, must first pass through the unloaded functional progression prior to working on kicking skills. Only after completing cutting and pivoting drills off the involved lower extremity are these athletes ready to begin kicking.

If a football kicker is a soccer-style kicker, all kicking in the functional progression program should be done soccer-style. If the kicker kicks from a straight approach, all kicking in the program should be from straight approach. The kicker's specific number of steps when approaching the ball should also be used. If the kicker uses a one-step approach, this is the manner in which kicking should be stressed. Although this is a rare problem (unless you are kicking outdoors in subfreezing weather), if the regulation ball is too heavy or not conducive to the practice setting, a foam rubber ball can be used. Place kickers may also use custom nets set directly in front of the ball. The portable net apparatus is made specifically for catching a regulation ball kicked with 100% effort.

Kicking at other than full velocity is difficult to perform and may even create abnormal kicking mechanics. Gradually increasing the kicking distance is a better way to assist the kicker in grasping the idea of gradually regaining preinjury kicking distance. For example, if preinjury kicking distance was 60 yards, then initial efforts might center on a distance of 30 yards. Work should continue here, stressing at least half the number of kicks performed in a practice setting prior to injury. When the number of kicks has been increased to preinjury level, distance can be increased, again gradually building up to the desired number of kicks.

Soccer players should progress kicking drills in a similar fashion. Efforts early on should focus on simple ball handling and juggling drills. These activities should be progressed to jogging drills with the soccer ball. As in the unloaded segment of functional progression, the athlete should be eased back into acceleration, deceleration, and pivoting maneuvers. Although the athlete at this point in the program has already advanced through the figure-eight and cutting sequence, ball handling in this way has not been stressed. Early unloaded efforts demanded concentration on the figure-eight and cutting drills. Now you are asking the athlete to remove the conscious mind from these activities and concentrate on handling the soccer ball. As these skills are mastered, jogging can be progressed to three-quarter speed sprinting and finally to sprinting with the ball. As you learned in the unloaded phase of functional progression, once full-speed drills at longer distances are conquered, the distance can be shortened to make the angle of cutting more acute.

Goal Play

The goal keeper must exhibit all basic functional progression skills as found in the unloaded section. In addition, loaded skills must be stressed, as this position involves forceful falls on the ground or ice and occasional encounters with players moving at high speeds toward the goal.

Skills inherent to the goal keeper position involve redirecting or blocking an incoming shot and then passing, throwing, or kicking the ball to a teammate. The soccer and team handball goal keeper must rely on the bare hands to clutch an incoming shot. After upper extremity injury, it is a good idea to use a softer ball in initial catching efforts. You or a teammate should stand 8 to 10 feet away from the goal keeper and toss the ball at half speed directly to the patient. The degree of difficulty can be increased by throwing the ball to the patient's right or left side, as well as making him or her jump for the ball. After upper extremity injury the athlete should have progressed through the unloaded phase of functional progression, including a graduated forward rolling sequence. You can make the task more difficult by throwing the ball so that the athlete must dive to make the catch, absorbing the force of the fall. As previously discussed, additional padding of the area may initially be required. When this drill has been mastered, a quicker response on the goal keeper's part can be stressed by increasing the speed of the incoming ball, decreasing the distance of the shot, or by decreasing the length of time between shots. After completing this phase, "live" shots from teammates may be introduced.

Hockey and lacrosse goalies often must perform in the same manner as the soccer goalie, frequently diving after loose pucks or balls. These athletes can be progressed in the same manner as just described. Another prime concern at this stage is the athlete's ability to react to one shot and quickly react to another incoming shot from a rebound. To prepare the goal keeper for such circumstances, repetitive shots from more than one teammate with little or no recovery time between shots is a practical drill.

♦ Summary

In the ideal functional progression program the recuperating athlete is exposed to every potential game situation in a controlled environment before returning to competition. This should be your goal, especially with athletes who participate in collision and contact sports. In such sports strange and unforeseen instances often arise, and it is difficult to prepare the athlete for every one of them. But it is your duty to break down the activities the athlete must perform on returning to competition and safely progress the player through them. If you do not, you leave the athlete with insecurities and unanswered questions. If you do, the athlete will be ready for a safe return to the high demands of contact and collision sports.

At the beginning of this chapter, Table 4.3 gave you an idea of the functional progression for athletes involved in contact and collision sports. Now, with an in-depth understanding of the skills inherent to each of these steps, you can refer back to it as a checklist to use as your athlete conquers each phase of the functional progression program.

CHAPTER 5

♦♦♦

Combat Sports

Combat sports are those sports where the prime objective is to exert superior physical force over an opponent in an effort to gain an advantage. They emphasize strength, quickness, agility, and anaerobic endurance. Popular combat sports are boxing, wrestling, judo, tae kwon do, karate, and other forms of the martial arts. These sports are similar to contact and collision sports in that physical contact is an inherent part of the sport. But some combat sports take this contact one step further. In collision and contact sports, physical contact is allowed to gain an advantage over an opponent in a team sport setting. In combat sports, the actual purpose is to render opposing players incapable of defending themselves. Judo players attempt to control their opponents and "throw" them to the mat. Wrestlers attempt to control and pin the opponent's shoulders to the wrestling mat. Subsequent physical control gained over the opponent is then rewarded by a sport-specific point system.

Protective devices are used in most combat sports. Boxers wear gloves, most wrestlers wear head gear, and tae kwon do participants wear elaborate protective padding. Judo and karate participants use no protection. Whether protection is used or not, injuries occur. Since there is significant contact and to a lesser degree collision between opponents, the type of injuries seen are similar to those in contact and collision sports (see Table 4.1 on page 48).

Rehabilitation guidelines for combat sports are also similar to those found in chapter 4 for collision and contact sports. Refer to Table 4.2 on page 48 for these rehabilitation concerns. As with collision and contact sports, other acute incidents may occur during combat sports unlike those commonly seen in rehabilitation. Unconsciousness, acute orthopedic trauma (fractures and dislocations), facial lacerations, and similar conditions are not within the scope of this book.

For our purposes, we'll divide combat sports into two categories: those that involve striking the opponent and those that do not. Striking can be done with the arms or legs. Kicking and/or striking an opponent is common in such sports as boxing, karate, tae kwon do, and other forms of the martial arts. The combat sports that do not allow striking the opponent certainly involve physical contact, but striking and kicking are not legal functions of the sport. Sports in this category are wrestling and judo. As the two types of combat sports are inherently different, functional progression for them must be different as well. The rest of this chapter deals with functional progression programs for striking and nonstriking combat sports.

♦ Striking Functional Progressions

As we discussed in chapter 4 for collision sports, the major emphasis in functional progression for combat sports should be on force delivery and force acceptance. Ability to generate force directed at the opponent and to adequately dissipate force from the opponent is even more important in combat sports than in collision sports. Greater importance is placed on these areas because

• physical contact is the main component of combat sports,

• force delivery and force acceptance are often required in abnormal or inefficient body postures, and

• the failure to adequately protect oneself may lead to serious injury.

For these reasons, you must stress the importance of an adequate strength base, sufficient aerobic, anaerobic, and musculoskeletal endurance, as well as proprioception and balance.

All combat sport athletes need to proceed through the unloaded functional progression program after lower extremity or upper extremity injury. Unloaded activities will ready the athlete to carry out sport-specific functions with relative ease. Just as American-football players begin with footwork skills specific to their positions, boxers and karate or tae kwon do participants begin with unloaded activities particular to their functions. Frequently, activities that stress proper form are done repeatedly during training for these sports. Stressing not only proper foot position but overall body posture and correct form to deliver a block or punch, these activities are routinely performed time after time in practice. Boxers frequently incorporate such activities into normal training regimes. Fighting an imaginary opponent stresses not only proper form but also speed and the anaerobic energy systems. As soon as the athlete is able, these sport-specific activities should be incorporated into the program. Once isolated individual activities present no difficulty for the athlete, he or she can move on to sparring with a partner. If you are knowledgeable in the specific sport, feel free to be the sparring partner yourself. If you are not, have a coach or fellow athlete help. No contact should be allowed during initial sparring. Instead the athlete practices attacking and defending skills, with no blows landed. It requires self-control to move authentically while refraining from contact.

Mock combat and sparring activities are helpful; however, you must place greater importance on a loaded functional progression program before allowing the athlete to return to activity. The best way to prepare your combat sport participants to return to full activity is via controlled combat drills that involve punching and kicking (force delivery) and blocking or receiving blows (force acceptance).

If protective equipment is worn in the striking sport it should also be worn during loaded functional progression drills. Emphasize correct form during punch or kick delivery and optimum body position to receive the punch or kick. The trunk, hips, and knees should remain slightly flexed over a stable unilateral or bilateral base of support as the athlete performs these drills.

Lower Extremity

As a stable base of support is required to successfully strike an opponent and to ward off incoming blows, it stands to reason that the lower extremities play an important role in combat sports. It also makes sense that the lower extremity is often injured in combat sports. Let's move on to discuss specific activities to incorporate into your functional program following lower extremity injury.

Loaded Activities

Because combat sports involve direct participation with another individual, functional progression activities should involve a partner as early as possible. In most combat sports, established weight classifications match athletes of approximately the same weight against one another. To minimize the chance for reinjury during the loaded phase of functional progression you should use these weight classifications to allow athletes of the same approximate weight to work together. Somatotype should also be considered. The length of the arms and legs are important factors in one's ability to strike an opponent. Try to match ectomorphs with ectomorphs and mesomorphs with mesomorphs.

Combat sport competitions are usually divided into time periods in the neighborhood of 2 to 3 minutes. Depending on the sport, the competition varies in the number of 2 to 3 minute periods. Perform functional progression drills for sport-specific durations. As with running, jumping, and other activities, you will have to gradually ease the combat athlete back into normal playing time frames. For example, if the wrestler you are working with needs to return to 3 periods of 2 minutes, you may need to start at 1 minute and gradually progress to 2 minutes.

Lower extremity work is minimal during upper extremity force delivery activity. Upper extremity striking activities as they relate to lower extremity functional progression should stress adequate form and sufficient follow-through. Careful attention should be directed at proper base of support and symmetrical weight shift. The combat sport athlete should use both upper extremities to deliver force, thereby loading both the lower extremities to provide stability.

Force delivery.   Kicking of course involves significant lower extremity activity. One leg is required to deliver the force quickly and accurately. Simultaneously, the opposite leg must be strong enough to support body weight (see Figure 5.1).

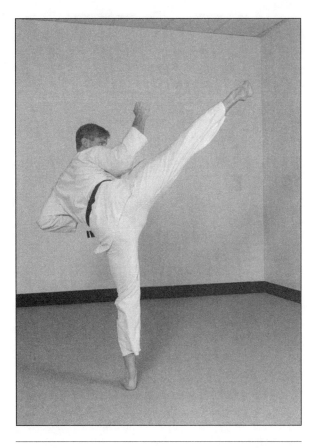

Figure 5.1 A stable base of support is required for combat sport force delivery (kick), and force acceptance (blocking kick) emphasizes trunk, hip, and knee flexion over a stable unilateral or bilateral base of support.

Adequate flexibility, strength, and proprioception are absolute musts for both legs after lower extremity injury.

Initially, shadow kick-boxing is an excellent activity. Require the athlete to perform single repetitions using both the involved and noninvolved leg. Early work is on controlled performance at half normal speed. As form and accuracy improve, increase speed to three-quarters normal and finally to full velocity. A rule of thumb is to allow kicking activities for half the total time required in real competition. This can be followed by three-quarters of the total time and finally a return to full-length competition times.

When stressing kicking drills with the involved leg, use additional padding to ease into contact drills. Many kicking sports allow soft protective padding for the feet during practice, and some allow this protection during competition. During the functional progression program, this extra padding is encouraged. When such footwear is disallowed or unavailable, consider using padded kicking targets. Heavy yet soft stationary dummies may be used for such kicking drills. These stationary targets are easily struck and offer sufficient padding for the involved lower extremity.

Force acceptance. Force acceptance requires a sound base of support to adequately dissipate force and to evade incoming blows. As with the force delivery series, work on force acceptance should be performed for sport-specific times. A special area of concern regarding force acceptance by the lower extremities is unilateral or off-balance work. Initially, force acceptance by the lower extremity should be done with symmetrical weight bearing and a solid base of support. Feet should be shoulder-width apart, with the hips and knees flexed slightly. As efforts here become easy, ask the athlete to narrow the base of support by standing with the feet together. Initially allow the hips and knees to be flexed slightly. However, once the athlete performs well in this position, progress to no hip and knee flexion. This will elevate the center of gravity and subsequently make standing more difficult. Work can then be progressed to off-balance efforts and single-leg stance activities.

Use moderation as the recuperating athlete accepts incoming forces. At the outset, blows directed at the athlete must be at half speed and half force. Progress gradually to full speed and full force for punches and kicks. Also, in the beginning the athlete should be fully aware from which direction the incoming blow is coming. Once full-speed and full-force blows are absorbed without difficulty, you can begin unexpected blows. Again, these unexpected blows must be at half speed and force initially and gradually advanced as the athlete tolerates.

If protective equipment over the injured area is allowed by the rules governing the sport, this equipment may be used in the functional progression program. However, if protective equipment is not allowed over the injured area, using protection during functional progression may be contraindicated. The recuperating athlete must be physically and mentally ready to accept physical contact. If the individual is overly concerned about the ability to accept force at the injured area, this phase of functional progression is premature.

Upper Extremity

Adequate upper extremity function is a must in striking combat sports. The athlete must be able to strike an opponent effectively with either arm and block incoming blows with either arm. Let's look at the basic principles governing functional progression for the combat sport athlete following upper extremity injury.

Loaded Activities

Most of the work required of the upper extremity during combat sports is force delivery. Therefore, the combat athlete recovering from an upper extremity injury must be able to deliver force with and accept force on the involved arm. If protective padding is allowed, you may wish to pad the involved arm for force acceptance drills. If protective padding is not used in the sport, you must ready the athlete without the assistance of extra padding. The same principles apply to accepting force with the injured arm as to accepting force with the injured leg. Progress with moderation. Refer to page 65 for specifics.

Force delivery is a vital upper extremity function in combat sports. The boxer or karate participant unable to strike the opponent with the arms is of no threat to an opponent. Punches must be fluid and quick. To score points, punches must be accurate as well. Punches that strike the opponent may be thrown one at a time or in succession (combination punches). The athlete must deliver punches quickly while at the same time defending punches from the opponent. It is to the athlete's advantage to be able to throw a punch while the opponent is punching (a counterpunch; see Figure 5.2).

Single punching.   Functional progression drills must first stress isolated, singular punching at stationary inanimate objects (or at a well-protected partner who is not allowed to strike back). These activities are followed by combination punching drills and, finally, counter-punching drills.

Initial emphasis is placed on proper upper extremity form. Again, shadow boxing is often beneficial during this phase. Throwing single punches at an imaginary opponent should be performed with a sound base of support. The trunk and knees should be flexed slightly, and the feet should be slightly greater than shoulder-width apart. Singular blows, alternating between the involved upper extremity

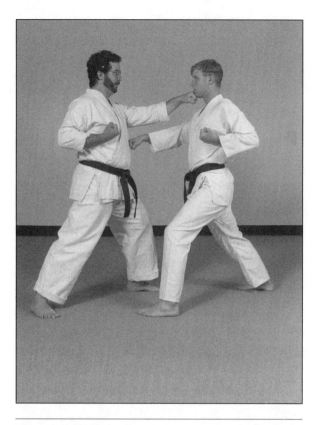

Figure 5.2   Accepting force with simultaneous force delivery (counterpunching).

and noninvolved side, should be performed. Begin with half the total competition time. Progress to the routine length of time and allow a sport-specific rest period. Ideally, these striking maneuvers should be performed with sport-specific footwork drills, also. Allowing the athlete to move in the competition arena as would be done during real competition stresses the cardiovascular and musculoskeletal systems. By combining lower extremity function with the upper extremity functional progression program, you also help to take the athlete's conscious mind off the upper extremity work.

Once single punches are easy for the athlete, counterpunches using the involved arm should be stressed. Stress different combinations, and you should assist with verbal instructions. Let's use an example of a karate participant who has sustained an acromioclavicular sprain. You can allow this athlete to pursue and evade an imaginary opponent throwing combination punches. Instruct the athlete to strike with the left arm, followed by the right arm, followed immediately by the left. Next, instruct the athlete to strike with the left arm, perform a shoulder roll, regain a stance, and strike with the left hand, followed by the right, followed immediately by two right-hand blows. There is no one best way to work on this. Emphasize quick movements with proper form, stressing immediate response to verbal instructions.

Counterpunching. Once the athlete has progressed satisfactorily to this level, you can begin working on counterpunching. For this activity, a coach or other person trained in the sport is helpful. This person throws punches at the recuperating athlete but does not make contact. The assistant is able to produce situations similar to competition, which requires the recuperating individual to react as she or he would in a real match. This activity should be as close to actual competition as is possible with no contact allowed. Once the athlete can perform these activities for competition-specific durations you can begin stressing the transition to contact punching.

Contact punching. Striking a stationary target is a great way to ensure that the combat athlete is ready to begin contact punching. A punching bag or a well-padded opponent is suitable for early force delivery through the affected upper extremity (see Figure 5.3). As you learned earlier in this chapter, moderation is the key. If the athlete has progressed readily to this point, he or she may be overzealous at this stage, wanting to deliver full-force and full-speed blows immediately. However, the same progression to full speed and full force with ample recovery time is vital.

♦ Nonstriking Functional Progressions

Combat sports that do not allow striking an opponent instead emphasize exerting physical control over the opponent. Points are awarded for various degrees of control. In wrestling, control is exhibited by the ability to grasp and throw the opponent to the mat or to dominate the opponent while on the mat. In judo, victory can result when one athlete throws the other squarely on the back onto the mat. The free-style wrestler is awarded victory when able to pin the opponent's shoulders to the mat.

As with striking sports, nonstriking combat athletes must possess strength, quickness, and good

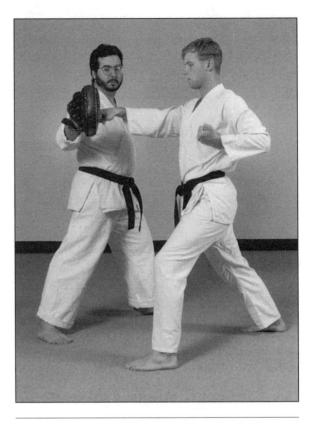

Figure 5.3 A stationary target is a good way to begin contact punching.

anaerobic fitness. In functional progression programs for the nonstriking combat athlete, emphasize

- bringing an opponent down to the mat (takedown drills),
- controlling oneself while being taken down to the mat,
- controlling the opponent while on the mat, and
- countering opponent's controlling maneuvers.

In our discussion of nonstriking combat sports, drills are referred to as being in the "up" position or in the "down" position. Drills in the up position refer to those in which both participants are standing on their feet. Drills in the down position refer to those in which both individuals are on the mat. Once again, activities will be classified as either force delivery or force acceptance drills. In nonstriking combat drills, force delivery in the up position refers to take-downs, whereas force acceptance refers to being taken down. When participants are down on the mat, force delivery refers to the athlete controlling an opponent, whereas force acceptance refers to being controlled by an opponent. Let's use wrestling as an example. Both athletes are up. Athlete A gains control and throw athlete B to the mat. Athlete A is involved in force delivery, while athlete B is involved in force acceptance. Once on the mat, athlete B reverses the situation and now has athlete A on his back about to be pinned. In this case, athlete B is involved in force delivery and athlete A in force acceptance.

As with all functional progression drills, stress the injured area gradually. For example, for an acromioclavicular sprain of the right shoulder, force delivery and acceptance should begin with activities in which the left arm can assist the right arm. Progression is to isolated use of the right arm. However, when control over an opponent is paramount, isolated upper or lower extremity function is not an efficient choice. Let's look at some of the specifics of a functional progression program for nonstriking combat athletes.

Down-Position Activities

With both participants on the mat, emphasis is on gaining and maintaining control over the opponent. Control is exerted over the opponent by keeping a legal, tight grasp and attempting to keep the opponent at a physical disadvantage. In the down posi-

tion, an athlete is either delivering the force and attempting to maintain the physical advantage or absorbing the force while trying to gain advantage over the opponent.

When two wrestlers are on the mat ready to begin competition, the down wrestler assumes a hands and knees position and the up wrestler positions over him (see Figure 5.4). Although these positions are not used in judo, the up and down positions are good foundations to build a functional progression program on. In the up and down positions, force delivery and acceptance skills are easily begun and progressed. If you do not have a sound working knowledge of the sport involved, a coach or a teammate of the recuperating athlete may be of great benefit.

Force Delivery

In down position activities, when the athlete is on the offensive, emphasize movements that control the opponent. As in the case with up position efforts, both athletes should be well aware of each other's moves. Initially, the uninjured teammate should not resist the efforts of the recuperating participant. Slow, purposeful movements emphasizing proper form and execution should be the rule. Once the injured athlete can perform the required movements, shift emphasis to greater speed of move-

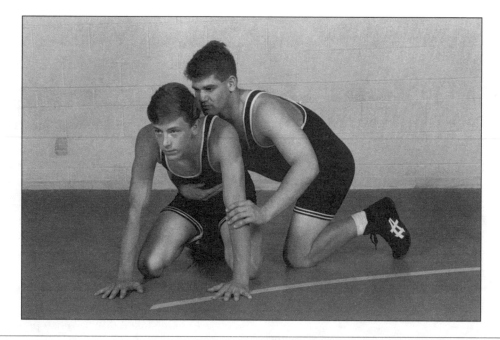

Figure 5.4   In wrestling, the defensive position stresses a compact quadruped position from which the athlete must quickly attempt to gain the offensive.

ment. Repetitive drills should be stressed in which you or another trained observer watch for substitutions for desired movements. Possible positions the individual may assume are numerous. Some positions may reproduce the initial mechanism of injury or be otherwise dangerous to the recuperating individual. You must ensure that the athlete can assume all positions in a controlled way without encountering resistance from the opponent. Then and only then will you allow the opponent to offer resistance. Once the opponent is allowed to offer resistance, you can begin to work the recuperating athlete for durations comparable to competition. Remember to begin with shorter periods of time and progress to regulation time as tolerated by the athlete. Allow adequate rest periods.

Force Acceptance

In nonstriking combat sport, participants must be able to withstand the positions in which the opponent exerts physical control. Often these positions will place a recuperating athlete at risk for reinjury. Therefore, prior to working with a teammate acting as an opponent, the recuperating athlete must be able to assume the positions in which he or she is controlled. Working with the coach or another well-informed participant, the injured individual should be placed in positions without extraneous resistance. Unloaded activities are absolutely vital prior to beginning loaded work. These precarious positions are potentially dangerous and should be well supervised.

When the nonstriking combat athlete is in a down position on the mat and the opponent is delivering force, the athlete on the receiving end of the force has two options: to counter the force with a move to attain an advantage over the opponent, or to escape from the situation. Functional progression drills should ready athletes for both options.

Escape

Nonstriking combat sports teach fundamental ways to escape situations in which an individual is being controlled. Functional progression drills should address these escape moves. Again, initial emphasis is on slow, purposeful movements to reinforce proper form and execution. When these activities are easy for the athlete, the degree of difficulty is increased as well as the speed with which the drill is performed.

Countermovements

Because the chief objective in nonstriking combat sports is to control the opponent, and not to run away, the athlete must eventually try to regain dominance of the opponent. Working with a teammate of the same weight, the recuperating athlete should be informed of every move the teammate will perform. This will allow the athlete to react to a known stress prior to being placed at a physical disadvantage. As with all functional progression drills, simple tasks should precede the more difficult maneuvers. Therefore, simple countermoves should be stressed from which the individual can move from a disadvantage to a physical advantage. A thorough understanding of the nonstriking combat sport is necessary, or you should work along with the coach to ensure that proper technique is used.

Once the athlete is able to gain the physical advantage over a passive teammate, the teammate should now provide opposition to the athlete's actions. The recuperating individual should still be fully informed of the intended actions of the teammate. However, the speed of the action should now be gradually increased to competitive levels.

Up-Position Activities

Usually, the nonstriking combat athlete in the up-position is best suited to deliver force. However, while in this position the athlete must be aware of the opponent's countering and escape moves. Let's take a look at the functional progression drills for the up-position nonstriking athlete.

Put simply, the objective of both participants in up-position activities is to take the opponent to the mat. During this attempt to take the opponent down, it is vital to maintain control. To maintain control, a firm grasp of the opponent must be secured and held during the fall to the mat. As you can see, potential injury is a real concern for the athlete being controlled. However, with the athlete in control focusing on maintaining the opponent under control, the potential for injury during the fall is also very real for the controlling athlete. For our purposes, force delivery will be synonymous with control, and force acceptance will mean being controlled. Functional progression drills must be geared toward the safe return to force delivery and force acceptance.

As functional progression efforts in the up position are really controlled falls, care must be taken to minimize chances for reinjury. Combat athletes should be matched according to weight. (As this is common for wrestling and judo, finding opponents of the same approximate weight should not be a problem.) Remember that when possible the recuperating athlete should be matched with a teammate of the same somatotype. When feasible, initial efforts in the functional progression program may be performed with a teammate one weight class under the recuperating athlete's class. If this is to be done, keep in mind the potential harm to the lighter teammate and the psychological effects on both individuals. Make sure that the lighter teammate understands the importance of assisting the recuperating athlete. The lighter teammate should not be made to feel he or she is an object for physical abuse, and the recuperating athlete should not feel belittled for competing against a lighter opponent.

Adequate padding should be used for this phase of the program. Additional soft padding in the form of extra mats may also be worthwhile. Protective equipment may be used if allowed by the sport. Make sure that ample space is provided for the drills. If possible, the entire mat area used for competition should also be utilized for functional progression. This will clear the area and reduce the risk of teammates falling on each other.

Force Delivery

Force delivery in the up position refers to the recuperating athlete taking down the opponent. You need to make sure that both participants understand what will happen. Both athletes must know the force delivery move the recuperating athlete will use. And both must know which force acceptance moves will be used to counter the force delivery move. As discussed on page 65, initial efforts should be performed at a walk-through pace in which proper positioning and form are stressed. These drills must also be performed straight on, so the athlete can see the opponent at all times. Drills should be progressed from simple to complex in terms of potential for reinjury. For example, the first walk-through drills should stress take-downs from a tall kneeling or kneeling position (see Figure 5.5a) prior to full-standing drills (Figure 5.5b).

Once stationary standing drills are completed without difficulty, speed may be increased to that of

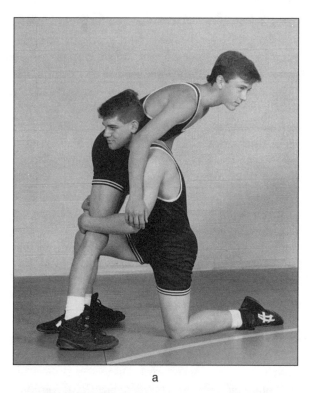

a

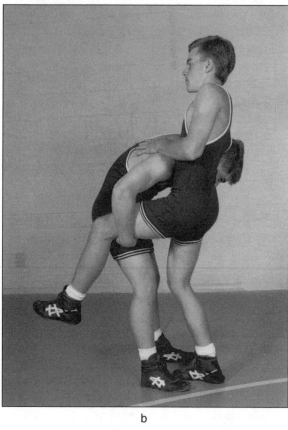

b

Figure 5.5 In wrestling or judo, the athlete tries to gain the offensive and take the opponent down to the mat. Forces can be progressed by beginning from (a) tall kneeling position and progressing to (b) standing take-down.

normal sport performance. Repetition of the skill is necessary to make the function more automatic and less of a conscious activity. A trained observer watching for abnormal substitutions by the athlete helps to ensure that bad habits are not created. These drills can be gradually progressed to full speed. A versatile athlete will have a full repertoire of take-down drills available, and all of them should be stressed in controlled fashion prior to actual competition.

Once full-speed drills from a head-on fashion present no problems, you can start the athlete on more aggressive challenges. Allow the opponent to move in an attempt to evade force delivered by the recuperating athlete and to counter the take-down moves. The opponent should still not be allowed to deliver force to the recuperating individual. These efforts more closely resemble actual competition, and time frames for competition may now be employed. Have the athlete attempt to take down a resisting opponent for time periods half that of normal competition. Duration can be gradually increased to competition standards, allowing adequate recovery time between sessions.

Force Acceptance

Fundamentals governing the functional progression for force acceptance are the same as those in force delivery. Moderation and a controlled return to full-speed function should be the rule. Even though the athlete is now being taken down, there should be no undue anxiety as he or she is fully aware of what the opponent will be doing. As with force delivery, force acceptance drills should progress from kneeling and tall kneeling take-downs to standing take-downs. Because the athlete is being thrown onto the mat, it may be important early on in the program to use extra padding. Efforts should begin from straight on and progress to those in which the athlete is not as readily able to see the opponent. Do not forget that some force delivery positions when the athlete is in the up position may involve being grasped and taken down from behind. This should not present a great amount of concern as long as the athlete knows what to expect. Early emphasis should be placed on readying oneself for contact with the mat. Once this presents no physical or psychological problems, the athlete is now ready to offer resistance to the opponent delivering the force.

◆ Special Concerns

Within our discussion of combat sports a few special concerns need to be addressed. First of all, although the vast majority of activity in combat sports is loaded, you must not overlook the unloaded component of functional progression. The traditional unloaded program works well up to the figure-eight drills. In these drills, to ensure that the athlete can pivot and push off of the injured lower extremity, you may also wish to progress him or her through a cutting sequence. But there are unloaded sport-specific drills that the combat athlete uses routinely that should also be included in the functional progression program. For the boxer and martial arts participant, shadow boxing is one such activity. For the judo participant, simultaneous upper and lower extremity movement patterns must be stressed to satisfactorily complete a throw. The wrestler must be able to sit-out (see Figure 5.6a), as well as sprawl (see Figure 5.6b), in split-second fashion. Other activities such as the spin drill, dodging a swinging heavy bag, and countless others routinely part of many practice sessions should figure highly in the functional progression program.

Another special concern is the concept of selective overload. This was discussed on page 70, where a lighter teammate is used as an opponent for the recuperating athlete. This can work in the opposite manner, too. Once the athlete is performing well with an athlete of the same weight, progression can be made to a heavier opponent. Caution must certainly prevail, but this can be a unique challenge for the recuperating athlete.

Finally, because these sports involve a good deal of physical contact, the resumption of activities should be systematic. The mechanism that caused the athlete's injury should be stressed again, but not until late in the program. It cannot be emphasized enough that the athlete must be able to assume all positions inherent to the sport prior to exposure to advanced activities.

◆ Summary

Combat sports are exciting, and those who play them are usually well motivated. The demands placed on combat athletes are significant, and returning these athletes to competition can be very

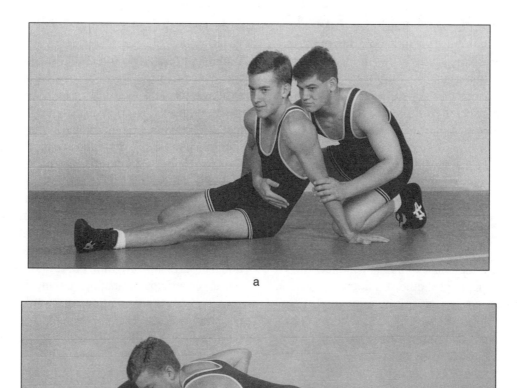

Figure 5.6   (a) The sit-out involves a quick move from the quadruped position to a seated position on the mat. (b) The sprawl involves a quick move from the quadruped position to a prone position on the mat.

rewarding. Keep in mind the basic functional progression program described in chapter 1 to provide a groundwork. Then add the specific activities presented in this chapter to prepare athletes to deliver and accept physical contact. A common-sense approach along with a program of increasingly graduated force delivery and acceptance drills will fully prepare your athletes for a safe return to combat sports.

CHAPTER 6

♦♦♦

Jump Training

As we have seen, specificity of training is important in determining the proper choice and sequence of exercise for sport training and the rehabilitation of athletic injuries. The movement of jumping is part of many sports activities, such as basketball, volleyball, gymnastics, and aerobic dancing. Running can be viewed as a repeated series of jump–landing cycles, so jump training should be included in the design and implementation of the overall training program.

It has generally been accepted that peak performance in sport requires both technical skill and power. In most activities skill is a combination of natural athletic ability and learned specialized proficiency. Success depends on the speed at which muscular force, or power, can be generated. Strength and conditioning programs usually have attempted to augment the force production system to generate maximal power. Because power is a combination of strength and speed, it will increase either through increasing the amount of work or force the muscles produce or by decreasing the amount of time taken to produce the force. Although weight training can increase strength, the speed of movement is more limited. The amount of time required to produce muscular force is an important variable for increasing the power output. *Plyometrics* is a form of training that attempts to combine speed of movement with strength.

Although the term *plyometric training* is relatively new, the concept itself is not. The roots of plyometric training are in eastern Europe, where it was known simply as jump training. The actual term *plyometrics* was coined by Fred Wilt, an American track and field coach (Wilt, 1975). The term's development is a little confusing. *Plyo* derived from the Greek word *plythein*, to increase, whereas *plio* is the Greek word for more. Both words could have been a basic prefix for plyometric. *Metric* literally

means to measure. The practical definition of plyometrics is a quick, powerful movement involving a prestretching of the muscle, thereby activating the stretch-shortening cycle. In other words, jump training takes advantage of the muscles' length-shortening cycle to increase power.

In the late 1960s and early 1970s, as the Eastern Bloc countries began to dominate sports requiring power, training methods became their focus. After the 1972 Olympics articles in coaching magazines began outlining a strange new system of jumps and bounds that the Soviets used to increase speed. Valery Borzov, the 100-m gold medalist, credited his success to plyometric exercise.

The Eastern Bloc countries were not the originators of plyometrics, however, just the organizers. American coaches had used this system of hops and jumps for years as a method of conditioning. Both rope jumping and bench hops were found to improve quickness and reaction times. The organization of plyometric training, however, has been credited to the legendary Soviet jump coach Yuri Verhoshanski who, during the late 1960s, began to organize these miscellaneous hops and jumps into a plan of training (Verhoshanski & Chornonson, 1967).

The main purpose of plyometric training is to heighten the excitability of the nervous system for improved reactive ability of the neuromuscular system (Voight & Draovitch, 1991). Any type of exercise in which the myotatic stretch reflex produces a more powerful response of the contracting muscle is plyometric in nature. All movement patterns in both athletics and daily activities involve repeated stretch-shortening cycles. Picture the jumping athlete as he or she prepares to transfer forward energy to upward energy. As the final step is taken prior to jumping, the loaded leg must stop the body's forward momentum and channel it upward.

As this occurs, the muscle undergoes an eccentric lengthening contraction to decelerate the movement and prestretch the muscle. This prestretch energy is then immediately released in an equal and opposite reaction, thereby producing kinetic energy. The neuromuscular system must react quickly to produce the concentric shortening contraction to prevent falling and produce the change in direction. Most elite athletes will naturally exhibit this ability to use stored kinetic energy. Less-gifted athletes can train this ability to enhance their production of power. Consequently, specific functional exercises that emphasize a rapid change of direction must be used to prepare patients and athletes for return to activity. Because plyometric exercises train specific movements in a biomechanically accurate manner, the muscles, tendons, and ligaments are all strengthened functionally.

◆ Principles of Plyometric Training

The goal of plyometric training is to decrease the time required between the yielding eccentric muscle contraction and the initiation of the overcoming concentric contraction. In the past, physiology of muscle contraction has focused mainly on the motor and stabilization roles of the muscular system. It is important to recognize, however, that the muscles also play an important role in shock absorption. This is especially true in jumping sports because the body must absorb the stress of landing. If the external force applied to the muscle overcomes its ability to resist, the muscle will lengthen. Lengthening occurs only after additional force is generated.

Normal physiologic movement rarely begins from a static starting position but rather is preceded by an eccentric prestretch that loads the muscle and prepares it for the ensuing concentric contraction. The coupling of this eccentric-concentric muscle contraction is known as the stretch-shortening cycle. The physiology of this stretch-shortening cycle can be divided into two components: the elastic properties of the muscle fibers and the proprioceptive reflexes. These components work together to produce a response, but they will be discussed separately to ease understanding.

Muscle Fibers

A muscle's mechanical characteristics can best be represented by a three-component model (Figure 6.1). A contractile component (CC), a series elastic component (SEC), and a parallel elastic component (PEC) interact with one another to produce a force output. Although the contractile component is usually the focal point of motor control, the series and parallel elastic components also play important roles in providing stability and integrity to the individual fibers when a muscle is lengthened. During muscle lengthening, energy is stored within the musculature in the form of kinetic energy.

When a muscle contracts concentrically, most of the force produced comes from the muscle fiber filaments sliding past one another. Force is registered externally by being transferred through the SEC (Figure 6.2). When eccentric contraction occurs, the muscle lengthens like a spring. With this lengthening, the SEC is also stretched and thereby allowed to contribute to the overall force production. So, the total force production is the sum of the

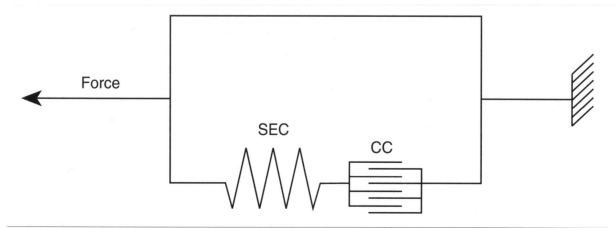

Figure 6.1 The three-component model of muscle behavior.

force produced by the contractile component and by the stretching of the SEC (Figure 6.3).

As an analogy, think of stretching a rubber band. When a stretch is applied, potential energy is stored and applied as it returns to its original length upon release.

Significant increases in concentric muscle force production when immediately preceded by an eccentric contraction have been documented (Asmussen & Bonde-Peterson, 1974; Bosco & Komi, 1979; Cavagna, Saibene, & Margaria, 1965). This may be due in part to the storage of elastic energy as the muscles are able to utilize the force produced by the SEC. When the muscle contracts concentrically, the elastic energy stored in the SEC can be recovered and used to augment the shortening contraction. The ability to use this stored elastic energy is affected by three variables: time, magnitude of stretch, and velocity of stretch (Enoka, 1988). The concentric contraction can be magnified only if the preceding eccentric contraction is of

short range and performed quickly without delay. Bosco and Komi (1979) proved this concept experimentally when they compared damped versus undamped jumps. Undamped jumps upon landing produced minimal knee flexion followed by an immediate rebound jump. With damped jumps, the knee flexion angle increased significantly. The power output was much higher with the undamped jumps. The increased knee flexion seen in the damped jumps decreased the muscles' elastic behavior, and the potential elastic energy stored in the SEC is consequently lost as heat. Similar investigations produced greater vertical jump height when the movement was preceded by a countermovement instead of a static jump (Asmussen & Bonde-Peterson, 1974; Bosco & Komi, 1982; Bosco, Tarkka, & Komi, 1982; Komi & Bosco, 1978).

Storage of elastic energy can also be affected by the type of muscle fiber involved in the contraction. Bosco (1987) noted a difference in the recoil of elastic energy in slow-twitch versus fast-twitch

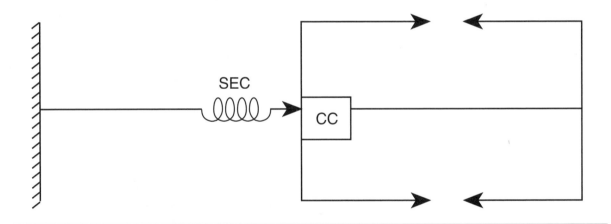

Figure 6.2   A concentric contraction.

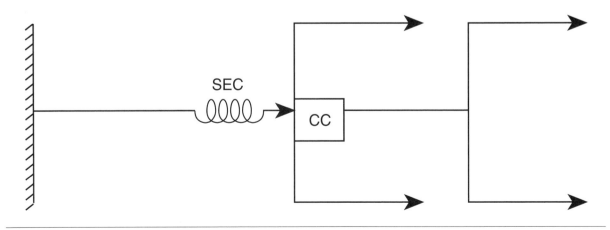

Figure 6.3   An eccentric contraction.

muscle fibers. This study indicated that fast-twitch muscle fibers respond to a high-speed, small-amplitude prestretch. The amount of elastic energy used was proportional to the amount stored. When a long and slow stretch is applied to muscle, slow- and fast-twitch fibers exhibit similar amounts of stored elastic energy; however, more of the stored energy is used by the slow-twitch fibers than by the fast-twitch fibers. This suggests that slow-twitch muscle fibers may be able to use elastic energy more efficiently in ballistic movement characterized by long and slow prestretching in the stretch-shortening cycle.

Proprioceptive Reflexes

The proprioceptive stretch reflex is the other mechanism by which force can be produced during the stretch-shortening cycle. Mechanoreceptors located in the muscles inform the CNS as to the degree of muscular stretch. The CNS then uses this information to influence muscle tone, motor execution programs, and kinesthetic awareness. The mechanoreceptors primarily responsible for the stretch reflex are the Golgi tendon organs (GTOs) and the muscle spindles (Lundon, 1985). Muscle spindles are complex stretch receptors located parallel within the muscle fibers. Sensory information regarding the length of the muscle spindle and the rate of the applied stretch is transmitted to the CNS. If the length of the surrounding muscle fibers is less than that of the spindle, the frequency of the nerve impulses from the spindle is reduced. When the muscle spindle stretches, an afferent sensory response is produced and transmitted by nerve fibers to the CNS. Neurological impulses are in turn sent back to the muscle, causing a motor response. As the muscle contracts, the stretch on the muscle spindle is relieved, thereby removing the original stimulus. The strength of the muscle spindle response is determined by the rate of stretch (Lundon, 1985). The faster the load is applied to the muscle, the greater the firing frequency of the spindle and the greater the resultant reflexive muscle contraction.

The Golgi tendon organ lies in the muscle tendon near where the muscle fiber attaches to the tendon. Unlike the facilitatory action of the muscle spindle, the GTO inhibits the muscle by contributing to a tension-limiting reflex. Because the GTO is in series alignment with the contracting muscle fibers, they become activated with tension or stretch within the muscle. Upon activation, sensory impulses transmitted to the CNS cause an inhibition of the alpha motoneurons of the contracting muscle and its synergists, thereby limiting the amount of force produced. During a concentric muscle contraction, activity of the muscle spindle is reduced because the surrounding muscle fibers are shortening. During an eccentric muscle contraction, the muscle stretch reflex generates more tension in the lengthening muscle. When the tension within the muscle reaches a potentially harmful level, the GTO fires, thereby reducing the excitation of the muscle. The muscle spindle and GTO systems oppose each other, and increasing force is produced. The descending neural pathways from the brain help to balance these forces and ultimately control which reflex will dominate (Rowinski, 1988).

The degree of muscle fiber elongation depends on three physiological factors. Fiber length is proportional to the amount of stretching force applied to the muscle. The ultimate elongation or deformation also depends on the absolute strength of the individual muscle fibers. The stronger the tensile strength, the less elongation to occur. The last factor influencing elongation is the muscle spindle's ability to produce a neurophysiological response. A muscle spindle with low sensitivity will have difficulty in overcoming the rapid elongation and will therefore produce a less powerful response. Plyometric training will assist in enhancing muscular control within the neurological system.

The increased force production during the stretch-shortening cycle is caused by the storage of elastic energy and the myotatic reflex activation of the muscle. The percentage of each component's contribution is unknown (Bosco & Komi, 1979). The increased amount of force production depends on how much time elapses between the eccentric and concentric contractions (Cavagna et al., 1965). This time frame can be defined as the *amortization phase* (Chu & Plummer, 1984), which is the electromechanic delay between eccentric and concentric contraction during which the muscle must switch from overcoming work to accelerating in the opposite direction. Komi (1984) found that the greatest amount of tension developed within the muscle during the stretch-shortening cycle occurred during the muscle lengthening phase just prior to the concentric contraction. This study concluded that an increased time in the amortization phase leads to a decrease in force production.

Physiologic performance can be improved by several mechanisms with plyometric training. While evidence has documented increased speed of the stretch reflex, the increased intensity of the subsequent muscle contraction may be best attributed to better recruitment of additional motor units (Chu, 1989). The force–velocity relationship states that the faster a muscle is loaded or lengthened eccentrically, the greater the resulting force output. Eccentric lengthening will also place a load on the elastic components of the muscle fibers. The stretch reflex may also increase the stiffness of the muscular spring by recruiting additional muscle fibers (Chu, 1989). This additional stiffness may allow the muscular system to use more external stress in the form of elastic recoil (Chu, 1989).

Another way plyometric training can increase force or power involves the inhibitory effect of the GTOs on force production. Because the GTO serves as a tension-limiting reflex restricting the amount of force produced, the stimulation threshold for the GTO becomes a limiting factor. Bosco and Komi (1979) have suggested that plyometric training may desensitize the GTO, thereby raising the level of inhibition. If the level of inhibition is raised, a greater amount of force production and load can be applied to the musculoskeletal system.

The last mechanism by which plyometric training may improve muscular performance concerns neuromuscular coordination. The speed of muscular contraction may be limited by neuromuscular coordination. In other words, the body may move only within a set speed range no matter how strong the muscles are. Training with an explosive prestretch of the muscle may improve the neural efficiency, thereby increasing neuromuscular performance. Plyometric training may promote changes within the neuromuscular system that allow the individual better control of the contracting muscle and its synergists. These changes could produce a greater net force even in the absence of morphological adaptation of the muscle. This neural adaptation can increase performance by enabling the nervous system to become more automatic.

In summary, effective plyometric training relies more on the rate of stretch rather than on the length of stretch. Emphasis should center on the reduction of the amortization phase. If the amortization phase is slow, the elastic energy is lost as heat, and the stretch reflex is not activated. Conversely, the faster the individual can switch from yielding eccentric work to overcoming concentric work, the more powerful the response.

♦ Program Development

Specificity should be the key concept of any training program. The individual's activities in daily living and in sport should be analyzed and broken down into components. To develop an athlete's plyometric program, begin by strengthening the body enough to withstand the large stress it will endure. Greater strength will result in greater force production due to an increased muscular cross-sectional area. Additionally, a larger cross-sectional area can contribute to the SEC and therefore to more stored elastic energy.

Plyometric exercises can be characterized as rapid eccentric loading of the musculoskeletal complex (Chu, 1989). This type of exercise trains the neuromuscular system by teaching it to better accept increased strength loads (Bielik, Chu, & Costello, 1986). By exploiting the stretch reflex, the nervous system's ability to react with maximal speed to the lengthening muscle may be improved, thereby increasing the maximal concentric force produced. Because plyometric training is attempting to remodel the neuromuscular system, all training programs should be designed with specificity (Rach, Grabiner, Gregor, & Garhammer, 1989). This will help to ensure that the body can accept the stress placed on it during return to function.

Prior to beginning a plyometric training program, a thorough study of the athlete's medical history, a structural examination, and a battery of functional tests should be performed to determine if any disqualifying condition exists. Eccentric muscle strength is important to plyometric training. Before allowing an athlete to begin a plyometric regime, a program of closed-chain stability training focusing on eccentric lower-quarter strength should be initiated. As discussed in chapter 2, open-chain strength training isolates a joint to single-plane movement. This, however, is not functional—we do not function sitting down. Closed-chain weight-bearing exercises allow the athlete to move functionally. Plyometric training can be considered a form of closed-chain exercise at the end of the stress continuum.

Once the athlete is cleared to participate in the plyometric program, initiate these safety precautions:

- Begin with an orthopedic screening evaluation.
- Develop an adequate strength base.
- Use supportive shoes.
- Use a resilient surface.
- Use a proper organized progression (SAID principle).
- Provide knowledgeable supervision to ensure proper technique.

Basic considerations when planning a plyometric training program are exercise intensity and athlete experience (Chu, 1992). Although plyometric training stresses the body to a high degree, it can be safe if initiated slowly into the overall conditioning program. Before you initiate a plyometric program, the athlete must have an adequate strength base. Poor strength in the lower extremities results in loss of stability upon landing and increases the stress absorbed by the soft tissues upon high impact forces. This results in reducing performance and increasing risk of injury.

The Eastern Bloc countries placed a one-repetition maximum in the squat at 1.5 to 2 times the individual's body weight before initiating lower-quarter plyometrics (Bielik, Chu, & Costello, 1986). Accordingly, a 200-pounder would have to squat 400 pounds before being allowed to begin plyometrics. Unfortunately, not many athletes meet this criteria. However, clinical and practical experience has demonstrated that plyometrics can be started without that kind of leg strength (Chu, 1992). Chu advocates a simple functional parameter to determine if an individual is strong enough to begin plyometrics. He recommends power squat testing using a weight equal to 60% of the individual's body weight. The individual is asked to perform five squat repetitions in five seconds. If he or she cannot perform this task, the program should return to emphasis on strength training until an adequate strength base is developed.

Flexibility Considerations

Due to the large amount of stress plyometric exercises apply to the musculoskeletal system, another important prerequisite for plyometric training is general and specific flexibility. All plyometric training sessions should begin with a general warm-up and flexibility exercise program. The warm-up should produce mild sweating (Jensen, 1975). The flexibility exercise should include both static and short dynamic movement patterns (Javorek, 1989).

Stability Testing

Stability testing prior to the initiation of plyometric training can be divided into two subcategories: static stability testing and dynamic movement testing.

Static Stability Testing

Static stability testing determines the individual's ability to stabilize and control the body. The muscles of postural support must be strong enough to withstand the stress of explosive training. Begin static stability testing with movements of low motor complexity and progress to difficult, highly complex skills. The basis for lower-quarter stability centers on single-leg strength. Difficulty can be increased by having the individual close his or her eyes. The basic static tests are one-leg standing and single-leg quarter squats held for 30 seconds. An individual should be able to perform one-legged standing for 30 seconds with eyes open and closed prior to the initiation of plyometric training. The individual should be observed for shaking or wobbling of the extremity joints. If more movement of a weight-bearing joint occurs in one direction than the other, the musculature producing the movement in the opposite direction needs to be assessed for specific weakness. If weakness is determined, the individual's program should be limited and emphasis placed on isolated strengthening of the weak muscles. Before beginning dynamic jump exercises, there should be no wobbling of the support leg during the quarter knee squats.

Dynamic Movement Testing

Dynamic movement testing assesses the individual's ability to produce explosive coordinated movement. Vertical jumping or single-leg jumping for distance can be used for the lower quarter. Russ Paine and Dr. David Drez (personal communication, 1992) have investigated the use of single-leg hopping for distance and as a determinant for return to sport following knee injury. A passing score on their test is 85% in regard to symmetry. The involved leg is tested twice and the average between the two trials is recorded. The noninvolved leg is tested in the same fashion, and then the scores of the noninvolved leg are divided by the scores of the involved leg and multiplied by 100. This provides the symmetry index score. In the upper quarter, the medicine ball toss is utilized as a functional assessment.

Plyometric Training

When the individual demonstrates both static and dynamic control of body weight with single-leg squats, plyometric training can be initiated. Plyometric training should consist of low-intensity drills progressed slowly and deliberately. As both skill and the strength foundation increase, moderate-intensity plyometrics can be introduced. Mature athletes with strong weight-training backgrounds can move immediately to ballistic-reactive plyometric exercises of high intensity (Chu, 1992).

Once an individual has been classified at a beginning, intermediate, or advanced level, a personalized plyometric program can be planned. Chu (1984, 1989) and Chu and Plumer (1984) have divided lower-quarter plyometric training into these six categories:

- In-place jumping
- Standing jumps
- Multiple response jumps and hops
- In-depth jumping and box drills
- Bounding
- High-stress sport-specific drills

♦ Plyometric Program Design

As with any conditioning program, the plyometric training program can be manipulated through four variables: Intensity, Volume, Frequency, and Recovery.

Intensity

Intensity is the amount of effort exerted. With traditional weight lifting, you can modify intensity by changing the amount of weight lifted. With plyometric training, intensity is instead controlled by the type of exercise performed. For instance, double-leg jumping is less stressful and therefore less intense than single-leg jumping. As with all functional exercise, plyometrics should progress from simple, low-intensity activities to complex high-intensity activities. Intensity can also be increased by altering a specific exercise. Adding external weight or raising the height of the step or box, for instance, will increase the exercise intensity.

Volume

Volume is the total amount of work performed in a single workout. With weight training, volume is recorded as the total amount of weight lifted (weight × repetitions). Volume of plyometric training is measured by counting the number of foot contacts. The recommended volume of foot contacts in any one session will vary inversely with the intensity of the exercise. A beginner should start with low-intensity exercise at a volume of 75 to 100 foot contacts. As ability increases, volume is increased to 200 to 250 foot contacts of low to moderate intensity.

Frequency

Frequency is the number of times an exercise session is performed during a training cycle. With weight training, exercise frequency is typically three times a week. Unfortunately, research on optimal frequency of plyometric exercise has not been conducted, so the best frequency for increased performance is not known. Chu (1992) has suggested that 48 to 72 hours of rest is necessary for full recovery before the next training stimulus. However, intensity plays a major role in determining the best frequency of training. If recovery is inadequate between sessions, muscle fatigue will result with a corresponding increase in neuromuscular reaction times. The beginner should allow at least 48 hours between training sessions.

Recovery

Recovery is the duration of rest between exercise sets. Manipulation of this variable depends on whether your goal is to increase power or muscular endurance. Since plyometric training is anaerobic, a longer recovery period should be used to allow restoration of metabolic stores. With power training, a work:rest ratio of 1:3 or 1:4 is recommended to allow for maximal recovery between sets. For endurance training, the work:rest ratio can be shortened to 1:1 or 1:2. Endurance training is typically a kind of circuit training, where the individual moves from one exercise set to another with minimal rest in between.

A plyometric program's success will depend on how well the four training variables are controlled, modified, and manipulated. In general, as the intensity of the exercise is increased, the volume should decrease. The corollary to this is as volume increases, intensity decreases. The overall key to controlling these variables is to be flexible and to listen to what the athlete's body is telling you. The body's response to the program should dictate the speed of progression. When in doubt about exercise intensity or volume, it is better to underestimate to prevent risk of injury.

♦ Plyometric Training Guidelines

As the plyometric program is initiated, the athlete must be informed of several guidelines (Voight & Draovitch, 1991). Deviation from these guidelines will result in minimal improvement and increased risk for injury.

• Plyometric training should be specific to the individual goals of the athlete. Activity-specific movement patterns should be trained. These sport-specific skills should be broken down and trained in their smaller components and then rebuilt into a coordinated activity-specific movement pattern.

• Work quality is more important than work quantity. Keep exercise intensity at a maximal level.

• The more intense the exercise, the greater the recovery time.

• Plyometric training may be of greatest benefit at the conclusion of the normal workout, when exercise under a partial to total fatigue environment specific to activity is best replicated. Only low- to medium-stress plyometrics should be done at the conclusion of a workout due to the increased risk of injury with high-stress drills.

• When proper technique can no longer be demonstrated, maximum volume has been achieved and the exercise must be stopped.

• The plyometric training program should be progressive. The volume and intensity can be modified in several ways.

   • Increase the number of exercises.

   • Increase the number of repetitions and sets.
   • Decrease the rest period between sets of exercise.

• Plyometric training sessions should be conducted no more than three times weekly in the preseason phase of training. During this phase, volume should prevail. During the competitive season, frequency should be reduced to twice weekly and intensity become more significant.

• Regular dynamic testing of the individual will provide important progression and motivational feedback.

Lower-Quarter Training

The beginning plyometric program should emphasize eccentric over concentric muscle contractions. Stress the relevance of the stretch-shortening cycle with decreased amortization time. Initiation of lower-quarter plyometric training begins with low-intensity, in-place jumps and multiple response jumps. Instruct the athlete in proper technique. The feet should be nearly flat in all landings and the athlete encouraged to "touch and go." (Think of landing on a hot bed of coals.) The goal is to reverse the landing as quickly as possible, spending a minimal amount of time on the ground.

Because the main concern with plyometric training is the intensity of the muscle contraction and the rate at which the resulting stretch-reflex action occurs, jump training from various heights is ideal. Depth jumps utilize the athlete's body weight and gravity to exert a force against the ground. The height of the box determines the intensity of the exercise and the response. This form of speed training was first described by Verhoshanski (1967), who analyzed different jump heights and determined that .8 meters was an ideal height for achieving maximum speed in switching from yielding to overcoming work. Maximal dynamic strength was achieved by dropping from a height of 1.10 meters.

Clinically, there has been disagreement about the optimal height for depth jumping. Lower box heights should be used with children and untrained individuals, whereas more experienced athletes can use a greater box height. Verhoshanski and Chornonson (1967) concluded that dropping from a height greater than 42 inches is counterproductive, as more time is spent in the amortization phase and the energy is lost as heat. Other Soviet researchers reported optimal results from a height of 320 centimeters (about 10 feet); however, they also reported that motivation was a problem and the risk of injury high (Dunsenev, 1982).

The chore of determining the proper jump height centers on the ability to achieve maximal height of the body's center of gravity following the depth jump. If the height of the box is too high, the legs spend too much time absorbing the force of impact upon landing and cannot reverse the eccentric loading fast enough to take advantage of the series elastic component of the muscle and to initiate the stretch-shortening reflex.

Optimal box height can be determined by establishing the individual's standing vertical jump reach. The individual then jumps from a box height of 18 inches. The goal is to achieve the standing jump-reach score. If the individual achieves this, the box height can then be increased in 6-inch increments. This procedure is repeated until the individual cannot reach the standing jump-reach score. This is the height that becomes the optimal box height for jump training. If the individual cannot achieve the standing jump-reach score from the 18-inch height, he or she is not ready for jump training; instead, emphasize increased functional strength. Follow this practical progression with variation.

- Box drop—rebound for height
- Box drop—rebound for linear distance
- Box drop—rebound to another box
- Box drop—rebound vertically, spring upon landing
- Box drop—rebound linearly, sprint upon landing
- Repeat sequence with one-legged hops and at increasing box heights.

Determining Plyometric Training Heights

Although clinical success has been noted with plyometric training, scientific studies of plyometrics are limited. Because of the wide variety of research design and methodology, it is extremely difficult to draw specific scientific conclusions about the effectiveness of plyometric training.

Verhoshanski's early work (1969) found that depth jumps effectively improved speed strength. In Verhoshanski's program individuals trained twice weekly, each session consisting of 4 sets of 10 repetitions, for a total of 40 jumps. It has been suggested that additional loading (increased box height) or adding weight to the body enhances results. Verhoshanski recommended no additional loading, as this would only change the timing of the eccentric to concentric muscle contraction and thereby decrease the session's effectiveness.

Since Verhoshanski's early work, several others have attempted to determine optimal jump training heights. In a controlled study, Adams (1984) assessed both vertical and horizontal jumping following depth jump training and found no significant difference in results from various training heights. However, isometric leg strength was significantly increased in the group training at a 1.5-meter box height. Research by Katchajov, Gomgeraze, and Revson (1976) was similar to Verhoshanski's in that the .8-meter drop height was most effective in producing results. Asmussen and Bonde-Peterson (1974) determined that maximal vertical jump rebound height occurred following a drop of .4 meters. Bosco and Komi (1978) found the optimal drop height for rebound jumping to be .5 meters for females and .62 meters for males. The conflicting data in the literature is likely due to different methods and subjects used.

Other than Verhoshanski's initial recommendation of 4 sets of 10 depth jumps, little research has been done on the optimal number of sets and repetitions in the training session. Low-impact plyometric drills such as hopping and bounding can produce a positive training effect. Von Arx (1984) demonstrated that horizontal bounding of approximately 4 meters with the center of gravity elevated a minimum of .5 meters corresponded with the training effects of rebound depth jumps.

Verhoshanski encouraged developing a strong base of strength before initiation of plyometric training. Depth jump training should be used in conjunction with traditional strengthening techniques. The available research suggests it is wise to implement general strength training with low-impact vertical and horizontal plyometrics before initiating more stressful depth jumping.

♦ Summary

Although the effects of plyometric training are not yet fully understood, plyometrics remains a widely used form of combining strength with speed training to functionally increase power. Though the research is somewhat contradictory, the neurophysiological concept of plyometric training is based on a sound foundation. To be successful, a plyometric training program should be designed and implemented only after an adequate strength base has been established. The benefits of this type of high-intensity training can be achieved safely if the individual is supervised by a knowledgeable person using common sense and following the prescribed training regime. Because year-round training often results in boredom and lack of motivation, the successful plyometric program should use a variety of exercises. Continued motivation and an organized progression are key to success.

CHAPTER 7

◆ ◆ ◆

Running Activities

Virtually all sports require forward propulsion of the body toward a finite goal. Although some athletes wear skis or skates to move them forward, athletes of most sports use no extra assistance other than a special pair of shoes. All baseball players must run around the bases to score. Outfielders must also run to catch fly balls. A gymnast sprints down the runway approaching the vault or across the mat for a tumbling pass. Almost all positions in football and soccer require running.

In track meets, runners are placed into one of three categories: sprinters, intermediate runners, and distance runners. For our purposes here, we'll limit runners to just two categories: sprinters and distance runners. Sprinters we'll define as runners in nontrack sports who are required to sprint in that sport and track runners who compete in distances of 1 mile or less. Examples of the first type of sprinter are players of baseball, basketball, soccer, and other team sports. Because these sports also involve throwing, jumping, and kicking, they are discussed in other chapters as well. Here functional progression for a return to sprinting required for specific sports

will be presented. The track sprinter will also be discussed.

Distance runners we'll define as those who run distances over 1 mile. These runners may compete in high school or college track or in cross-country. They might run in amateur or professional races where distances range from 5 kilometers (3.1 miles) to a marathon (26.2 miles) or beyond. Some distance runners may never participate in a formal race, content to run for enjoyment and cardiovascular benefit.

A discussion of the biomechanics of running and sprinting is well beyond the scope of this book. But whether you are rehabilitating a world class sprinter or a recreational jogger, a general understanding of running and sprinting is required. Because the mechanics of running in competition and running for pleasure are similar, types of injuries seen in these runners are also similar. There are many excellent texts that thoroughly describe running biomechanics and running injuries. In Table 7.1 you will find common lower extremity injuries that affect runners. Also, when treating the injured runner, keep in

Table 7.1 Common Lower Extremity Running Injuries

Back	Hip	Ankle/foot	Knee	Lower leg
Low back pain	Trochanteric bursitis	Tarsal/metatarsal stress fracture	Patellofemoral pain syndrome	Tibial/fibular stress fracture
	Femoral neck stress fracture	Achilles tendinitis	Chondromalacia patella	Posterior tibialis tendinitis
	Iliopectineal bursitis	Sever's disease	Iliotibial band friction syndrome	Exertional compartment syndrome
	Gluteus medius strain	Blisters, bunions, bunionettes	Popliteus tendinitis	
	Hip rotator muscle strain	Tarsal tunnel syndrome	Distal hamstring strain	
	Upper hamstring strain		Pes anserine bursitis	

mind these factors that contribute to lower extremity overuse injuries:

- Muscle strength balance
- Inadequate muscle strength
- Muscle-tendon unit inflexibility
- Poor aerobic, anaerobic, and musculoskeletal conditioning
- Excess body weight
- Training errors (a too-sudden increase in mileage; excess mileage; altered running gait)
- Change in running surface
- Change of running shoes or improper footwear
- Anatomical abnormalities (genu varus/valgus; forefoot or rearfoot varus/valgus; hypermobile or hypomobile first ray; tibial torsion; femoral anteversion; patellofemoral joint abnormalities; leg length inequality; pelvic obliquity)

Most running injuries result from microtrauma. Continuous striding transmits ground reaction forces up the legs, pelvis, and low back. The greater the distance, the greater number of foot contacts with the ground, which increases the risk for overuse injury. Many of these overuse injuries (or stress–failure injuries, as they are also known) are preventable. Common overuse injuries sustained by runners along with rehabilitation concerns for these conditions can be found in Table 7.2. As you can see, almost all running injuries affect the lower extremity. Therefore, functional progression guidelines to follow will address the lower extremity only.

◆ Functional Progression for Distance Runners

You learned in chapter 1 that functional progression drills should begin as soon as adequate motion and strength are present and pain and swelling have been controlled. You also learned that functional progression drills complement formal rehabilitation efforts. A return to running is no exception to these basic principles. The injured runner who is able to bear weight on the affected lower extremity should stress normal weight-bearing activities. However, this is not the time to let the runner resume preinjury distances.

Maintaining Endurance

Deleterious effects of bed rest and immobilization are well known to the health care professional. And even when the runner is not required to curtail activities to the point of bed rest, decrease in normal running can cause deconditioning. Initial efforts in the formal rehabilitation program should be geared toward decreasing the potential effects of deconditioning. Because most running injuries involve the legs, there is no problem in stressing the upper extremities to maintain aerobic and anaerobic fitness of the runner. When rehabilitating the distance runner, your emphasis should certainly be on the aerobic energy system. A customized upper extremity ergometer, such as the Biodex Upper Body Cycle,[1] provides an excellent workout (see Figure 7.1). If you do not have access to such a unit, a traditional bike or ergometer can be modified for upper extremity use. The traditional aerobic workout of 20 to 30 minutes at no less than 65% of maximum predicted heart rate is a good place to start, but remember that many distance runners are accustomed to aerobic work of much longer duration. You should incorporate the conditioning program as early as possible, attempting to approxi-

Table 7.2 Rehabilitation Concerns for Running Injuries

Body area	Rehabilitation concern
Low back	Adequate hamstring flexibility Pelvic and leg length symmetry Adequate abdominal, paravertebral, gluteal, and latissimus muscle strength Sound foot mechanics Activity modification
Hip	Adequate hamstring flexibility Pelvic and leg length symmetry Adequate hip rotator strength and flexibility Sound foot mechanics Activity modification
Knee	Adequate hamstring and calf flexibility Proper quadriceps:hamstring strength ratio Adequate iliotibial band flexibility Sound foot mechanics Activity modification
Ankle/foot	Adequate calf flexibility Sound foot mechanics Activity modification

[1]Biodex, Shirley, New York.

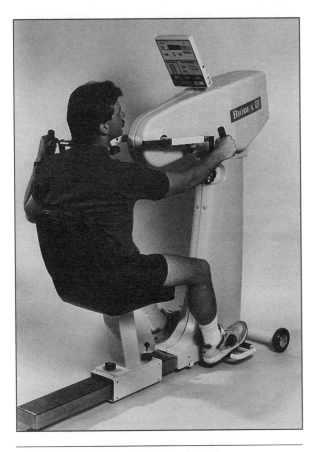

Figure 7.1 The Biodex Upper Body Cycle.
Courtesy Biodex Medical.

Table 7.3 Alternate Conditioning Activities

Weight-bearing status	Activity
None	Swimming
	Deep pool running with floats
Partial	Stationary cycling
	Rowing machine
	Pool walking
	Underwater treadmill walking
	Zuni Unloader
Full	Treadmill walking/running
	Minitramp running
	Rope jumping
	Cross-country skiing simulators
	Stair steppers

mate the normal aerobic training time to which the runner is accustomed.

Introduce other methods to elevate the physiologic loads as lower extremity status allows. When feasible, progress from nonweight-bearing to partial weight-bearing, and ultimately to full weight-bearing activities. Refer to Table 7.3 for suggested ways to stress the cardiovascular system as the lower extremity becomes able to accept increasing loads. When considering any of the alternate activities to improve aerobic conditioning, keep in mind that the runner must be both physically and psychologically comfortable with the training device and activity. Most importantly, never stress the injured body part beyond its capacity to protect itself. If the injured area is painful with activity or more swollen or painful after finishing activity, the runner's efforts are overly aggressive.

Returning to Running

Once the runner can bear full weight on the involved lower extremity with no pain and no limp, you may begin a return to running. To increase blood flow to the lower extremities before running, a warm-up that causes no pain at the injured area is recommended. Gentle stretching of the muscles of the back and lower extremities should follow. Give special attention to the injured muscles or the musculature surrounding the injured body part. Again, initial distance should be no greater than one-third the distance the athlete was comfortable with prior to injury.

The running surface should be flat and smooth. Distance runners will usually have to put in at least some of their distance on the road; they should run on the softer asphalt of the road instead of the harder sidewalks. Good running habits should be maintained, such as keeping in the proper direction regarding traffic and switching sides of the road. When running on the track, the runner should also routinely switch direction.

Distance and Duration

Stress moderation and graduation. The distance runner may need ultimately to get back to running 20 minutes or longer (and may have in fact been biking or swimming for this duration during rehabilitation), but when you introduce running into the program, you need to start with a shorter time. Therefore, you will need to continue cross-training on the bike or in the pool to achieve total training time. Say, for example, you are working with a runner with plantar fasciitis who wants to get back to 30 minutes of running, but jogging for only 5 minutes on the treadmill causes pain. You should remove this runner from the treadmill and spend the remaining 25 minutes on a partial weight-bearing activity that is painfree.

A gradual return to activity is a must, so before you start the program you need to know what level the runner needs to return to. Activity level is usually expressed in duration or distance, intensity or pace, and frequency. *Duration* is the length of the run, usually expressed in time. (Duration may also be expressed in terms of distance by runners who know the distance at which they train and how long it takes them.) *Intensity* refers to how hard the athlete runs. A better way to look at this is the pace at which the runner functions. Pace refers to how long it takes to cover a given distance and is usually expressed as minutes per mile. A runner who covers 1 mile in 4 minutes and 30 seconds obviously runs a faster pace than the runner who takes 6 minutes per mile. Finally, *frequency* refers to the number of times the runner will run in a set time frame, usually expressed as days per week. Most competitive runners will run every day, as will many recreational runners. When training before the beginning of a competitive season, some runners will run more than once a day. Others prefer to run every other day or less.

You need to understand these parameters. By manipulating them, you can bring your distance runners back in a graduated fashion. A gradual progression is the best guarantee against reinjury. The most sensitive parameter to adjust is duration. To start with an effective duration, you need to know how far, how often, and how hard the athlete was performing before the injury. Often, runners continue to run with pain; only when the pain affects performance do they seek medical attention. You will need to question your athletes carefully to ascertain when they started to run with pain. Once

you know the distance or duration at which symptoms began, a rule of thumb regarding initiating running is to start at no greater than one-third the distance or time that caused pain prior to injury.

You will need to use your judgment in assigning a beginning distance or time frame. Every case and every runner is unique. Be sure to consider how long the runner has been unable to run due to injury and the level of deconditioning. Needless to say, the longer the runner has been unable to run, and the poorer the level of preinjury and postinjury conditioning, the shorter the distances you should assign this runner initially.

When the athlete tolerates the initial distance without difficulty, distances may be gradually increased to preinjury levels. Progress in increments of one-fourth the total until the runner is able to perform a good 2-mile base. Once a distance of 2 miles is easily tolerated, allow half-mile increases. Let's look at an example to see these guidelines put into practice.

You are working with a recreational runner recovering from a tarsal navicular stress fracture. Your common goal is a return to running 4 miles three times a week at a pace of 7 minutes per mile. Throughout rehabilitation, this runner has been biking and swimming 45 minutes three times a week. How do you get her back on the street?

Because the distance is not that far, you should be able to safely begin at one-fourth of the preinjury status. Begin at 1 mile and let the runner perform that distance at least three or four times prior to increasing mileage. When the runner has tolerated 1 mile without difficulty, increase the distance to 1-1/2 miles. Let her run this distance at least twice before increasing the distance to 2 miles. When two runs of 2 miles are tolerated, increase the distance to

Table 7.4   Running Progression (4 miles every other day)

	Day 1	Day 2	Day 3	Day 4	Day 5	Day 6	Day 7
Week 1	1	0	1	0	1	0	0
Week 2	1-1/2	0	1-1/2	0	1-1/2	0	0
Week 3	2	0	2	0	2	0	0
Week 4	2-1/2	0	2-1/2	0	2-1/2	0	0
Week 5	3	0	3	0	3	0	0
Week 6	3-1/2	0	3-1/2	0	3-1/2	0	0
Week 7	4	0	4	0	4	0	0

2-1/2 miles, then to 3 miles, then to 3-1/2 miles, and finally to 4 miles. Remember, the runner must tolerate the same distance on at least two occasions before increasing mileage. Refer to Table 7.4 as a guide to use and modify.

Pace and Frequency

Are you finished with this runner once she has reached her goal of 4 miles? The answer is No—because you have not yet addressed running frequency or pace. Once the runner has reestablished a preinjury mileage base, pace and frequency can be addressed.

Initial efforts should begin at a comfortable pace. Once the desired mileage is no longer difficult, the runner can work on shaving time off the run. Perhaps it's best to have the athlete run a comfortable pace the first fourth of the run, increase to preinjury pace the middle half of the run, and use the last fourth to cool down. When the middle half of the run is not taxing, the athlete can begin the run at preinjury pace, maintain it for three-fourths of the total distance, and then use the last fourth to cool down. Finally the runner can run the entire distance at preinjury pace and add a brief cool-down after completing the desired mileage.

If you are working with an athlete who runs more than every other day, you still need to address running on back-to-back days. This should be done in a graduated manner. Initial efforts should be on regaining the preinjury mileage base. Once this is accomplished, the runner may begin putting daily workouts back to back. A good guideline is not to allow distances greater than half of the workout of the preceding day.

Let's use the case of a runner who needs to get back to running 4 miles every day. Once the 4-mile base is tolerated every other day, the runner can add a 2-mile workout on a day following a 4-mile run.

The next day, the regular 4-mile run is allowed followed by another 2-mile run. Now that this sequence has been tolerated, increase the 2-mile runs by half-mile increments until the runner reaches 4 miles. Remember—the runner must tolerate two sessions at an increased distance before you allow an increase in distance. See Table 7.5 for a quick reference to use and to modify.

Finally, you are ready to address running frequency. Unless the runner is taking part in early season workouts, running will be limited to once daily, so the functional progression program should also be performed once daily. If two running sessions are allowed, each scheduled daily workout must be cut in half. Other considerations include gradually progressing back into inclines, hills, and courses that may present treacherous footing.

This functional progression program may seem simplistic, but you need to progress the runner systematically. You should be familiar with your system and modify it according to special situations. Encourage constant feedback from the runner to prevent reinjury.

With the basic principles behind us, let's look briefly at a program for a return to sprinting.

♦ Functional Progression for Sprinters

The foundation for a return to sprinting has been laid in detail in the section on distance runners. Many of the same principles apply to the sprinter. The parameters that can be manipulated are virtually the same as for the distance runners, and, once again, moderation is the key.

Distances for true sprinting range from 60 feet down the baseball line to the 800-meter race. Team sports, however, often require the athlete to sprint shorter distances. In functional progression for

Table 7.5 Running Progression (4 miles daily)

	Day 1	Day 2	Day 3	Day 4	Day 5	Day 6	Day 7
Week 1	4	2	4	2	4	0	0
Week 2	4	2-1/2	4	2-1/2	4	0	0
Week 3	4	3	4	3	4	0	0
Week 4	4	3-1/2	4	3-1/2	4	0	0
Week 5	4	4	4	4	4	0	0

sprinting, we will look at basic guidelines that can be modified for any given sprinting distance.

Parameters to control in the sprinting functional progression are frequency and intensity. For sprinting, frequency is thought of in repetitions and sets, in addition to days per week. Intensity is more easily measured in the sprinter than in the distance runner. Intensity can be progressed by percentages of the full-speed sprint—that is, half-speed progressed to three-quarter speed and finally to full speed.

After an adequate warm-up and specific stretching of the injured tissue, the sprinter can begin to work on sprinting. The explosive start of a sprint is too strenuous to serve as a beginning point. Therefore, the sprinter is asked to begin the sprint from a standing position. As per our discussion of functional progression basics, a half-speed sprint refers to a jog, three-quarter speed refers to a half-speed sprint, and full-speed is full sprinting.

The total distance of the sprint is broken down into quarters. Let's use the 100-meter dash as an example. In getting the sprinter ready for the 100 meters, break the distance down to four intervals of 25 meters (see Figure 7.2). Initially, the sprinter should be able to jog the entire 100 meters without problems. After this is tolerated for at least two sets

of 10 repetitions, the program may be progressed. The next step is to jog the first 25 meters, then three-quarter speed sprint the middle 50 meters, and use the final 25 meters to slowly decelerate. When this is tolerated, the sprinter can jog the first 25 meters, perform a full sprint for the middle 50 meters, and again use the last 25 meters to slow down. Adequate rest should be allowed between the two sets of 10 repetitions. Stretching of the involved area is highly recommended between sets.

When the sprinter has adequately performed this first phase, efforts to begin from a sprint can be stressed. The sprinter should assume a normal starting position for the activity. For sprinters, it will be the 4-point stance. For the base runner attempting to steal, it will be a lead-off position (see Figure 7.3). And for the hockey player, it may be in the face-off position. Using our 100-meter sprinter as an example, initial efforts will begin from the stationary position and a three-quarter speed sprint will be performed from start to finish. When the desired distance has been completed for at least two sets of 10 repetitions, with adequate rest and stretching,

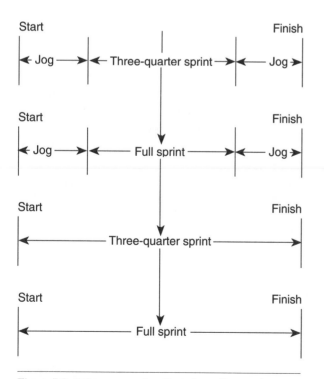

Figure 7.2   Distances can be adjusted to reflect requirements of the athlete's sport or activity.

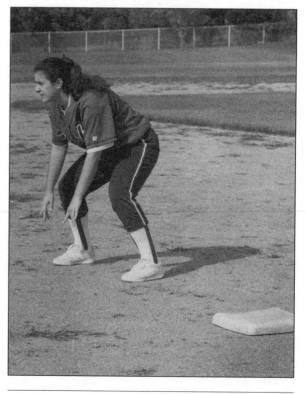

Figure 7.3   The stationary starting position for sprinting should be sport specific. One position the baseball or softball player should use is the lead-off position that emphasizes a quick crossover step of the inside foot.

full-speed sprinting is allowed from start to finish. These basic principles can be used for all athletes required to sprint in their sport. Once the athlete is comfortable with sprinting, noncontact sport-specific drills should begin. For example, at this stage the basketball player can dribble full speed the length of the court, and the tennis player can sprint full speed to the net.

♦ Summary

As you can see, the basic premise for a return to running and sprinting activities is no different from any other functional progression program. A graduated approach is a vital and fundamental guideline you must always adhere to. For runners and sprinters, break down the distance and manipulate duration, time, frequency, and intensity in a logical manner. This will send your running athletes back to their sport in top shape. You can easily apply these same principles to swimmers, cyclists, and other athletes involved in sprint or distance activities.

With the vast majority of sport activities behind us, let's turn our attention to athletes involved in throwing and overhead activities.

CHAPTER 8

◆◆◆

Throwing Activities

In the past 10 years we have seen a tremendous increase in the amount of information relating to shoulder pathology. The shoulder is a complex configuration made up of four joints to allow increased mobility. The *glenohumeral joint* is a minimally constrained articulation unique in its fine balance between mobility and stability. The glenohumeral joint has very little static or ligamentous stability. Passive static constraints that limit excessive translation include both osseus and fibrous tissue structures. The glenoid fossa is functionally deepened by the fibrocartilaginous labrum, which serves to increase the area of contact between the humeral head and the glenoid. The primary source of stability is dynamic and requires a unique synergism of all the muscles surrounding the shoulder. While the musculotendinous units of the rotator cuff provide some static restraint by acting as a barrier, their major function is their dynamic role in actively constraining the humeral head by compressing it into the glenoid. Any structural flaw in either the bony or musculotendinous units will result in a loss of perfect function. Injury occurring at any one of the four joints in the shoulder complex will disrupt and affect the others. Consequently, rehabilitation of the shoulder should include the entire kinetic chain.

◆ Repetitive Stress

An athlete's shoulder and elbow are exposed to various forces depending on his or her sport. The baseball pitch has been studied extensively in both clinical and laboratory settings. Comparison of many overhead activities has revealed that the throwing motion is fundamentally common to many sports. Examples include the tennis serve, the javelin throw, and the forward pass in football. Each activity presents its own specific problems depending on the stress and strain generated.

The majority of pathology seen in the upper quarter are overuse injuries. Repetitive microtrauma causes inflammation and eventually leads to soft tissue degeneration and breakdown. The most common presentation in the athlete's shoulder is pain and dysfunction. There is controversy about the exact cause of this dysfunction. The relationship among impingement, rotator cuff disease, and instability in individuals who repeatedly place their arm overhead has been debated. It is possible that subtle instability is responsible for the pain and dysfunction about the shoulder. During the throwing motion, the static stabilizers struggle in their attempt to control the stress placed on the shoulder. As a result, the humeral head translates, thereby stretching the capsule and stressing the glenoid labrum.

If these static stabilizers become damaged, the rotator cuff musculature must produce additional tension to control and limit the humeral head translation. This subtle instability should be regarded as a part of a continuum that eventually leads to impingement and rotator cuff disease. As the static stabilizers are stretched, increased glenohumeral translation occurs. In attempting to limit the translation, the rotator cuff works harder and eventually becomes fatigued. Tendinitis results, and tensile changes occur with tendon fiber failure. When this happens the rotator cuff can no longer control the humeral head and increased anterior-posterior migration of the humeral head occurs. The scapular rotators allow increased protraction, and impingement results. It becomes increasingly apparent that the shoulder joint is truly designed for mobility and only a delicate balance of forces provide it with passive and dynamic joint stability.

The act of overhead throwing imparts a great deal of repetitive stress on the upper quarter. The throwing motion is a highly complex dynamic process requiring multiple muscle synergy patterns. Synchronous firing of the dynamic rotator cuff muscles centers the humeral head in the most stable position within the glenoid. The scapular rotators also contribute by positioning the scapula for the best possible bony stability in the overhead position. This scapular movement occurs simultaneous with the humerus to maintain the balance and stability about the shoulder. Fatigue due to eccentric overload forces can complicate the thrower's shoulder, and breakdown begins to occur. Throughout the throwing motion, maximal stress is placed on the soft tissue structures. In many cases, these stresses are just below the maximal tolerance level of the structures. If these stresses are applied at a rate faster than the rate of tissue repair, or when the maximal level is exceeded, injury occurs. The synchrony of muscle firing is critical in achieving maximal function without injury. Any deficiency in either neuromuscular control or muscular strength and endurance will produce a significant and cumulative effect on shoulder function and increase the risk of injury. A shoulder performing at or near its physiological limitation without proper throwing mechanics, conditioning, or warm-up will eventually break down from overuse. The joints of the upper extremity most prone to injury from repeated throwing are the shoulder and the elbow.

Repetition of the throwing motion leads to gradual adaptive changes and hypertrophy of the soft tissue structures about the shoulder girdle. Minor alterations in the mechanics of the throwing motion, such as a prolonged wind-up phase, can lead to disruption of the balance between maximal stress and tissue tolerance. An understanding of biomechanics is very important in analyzing the throwing motion.

The Windup

The throwing motion begins with the preparatory or *wind-up* phase. The pitcher creates potential energy by drawing back on one leg and turning sideways. The conclusion of this phase occurs as the ball leaves the pitcher's glove. The cocking phase allows for proper arm and body positioning. It is during this phase that significant stress is placed on the anterior capsule and internal rotators of the shoulder. The shoulder is subjected to tremendous forces as the body rotates forward and the shoulder and arm lag behind. Momentum is transferred from the moving body to the throwing arm. It has been estimated that the force causing anterior translation at the glenohumeral joint is approximately 40% of body weight (Dillman, 1991). The contralateral leg is kicked forward and planted directly in front of the body. The energy produced by the trunk and lower extremities is transferred to the shoulder and arm. The cocking phase continues until the shoulder reaches maximum external rotation. The ball is not moved forward at all during this phase.

Acceleration

Acceleration starts with external rotation and abduction and continues until the ball is released. The body moves forward with the arm following behind. Angular velocity is estimated at 7000 to 8000 degrees a second at the shoulder and 3000 to 4000 degrees a second at the elbow (Dillman, 1991). Momentum from the body is converted into rotational movement at the arm. Acceleration concludes with ball release.

Follow-Through

The follow-through phase is where injury is most likely. In this phase the energy must be dissipated as body weight continues to transfer onto the contralateral leg. The deceleration forces are approximately two times greater than the acceleration forces and occur over a shorter time. Rapid shoulder internal rotation and abduction must be reduced to decelerate the arm. The distraction force acting on the glenohumeral joint during this phase is approximately 90% of body weight.

To propel a baseball with velocity and accuracy, the thrower must generate kinetic energy. Improper generation of kinetic energy results in overutilization of the muscular sources, causing injuries from fatigue and overuse. The act of throwing is not just arm motion but includes footwork, leg motion, and hip and trunk rotation. A tremendous amount of energy can be generated and released through the throwing arm. After the ball is released, this retained kinetic energy must be dissipated. Any improper transfer of energy, such as occurs in a shortened follow-through phase, can lead to injury. Disruption in any one of these areas can lead to uncoordinated movement, resulting in increased stress. Repetition of improper throwing motion leads to further trauma and injury.

♦ Rehabilitation

The increase in knowledge about shoulder pathology has led to an increased emphasis on injury prevention and early rehabilitation. Once an accurate diagnosis is made, aggressive rehabilitation should follow. Whereas most shoulder pathologies respond well to a nonoperative program, rehabilitation is crucial to success in the operative patient. Diagnosis dictates the type of rehabilitation program used. The specific rehabilitation program should be modified based on the individual's diagnosis, severity of injury, and functional expectations.

Phase One: Acute Management

Initially, emphasize the reduction of inflammation with rest and nonsteroidal, anti-inflammatory medications. "Rest" should be regarded as a relative term. "Activity modification" or "activity without abusive overload" are more accurate descriptions. Physical therapy modalities such as ultrasound and electrical stimulation can also be helpful in reducing inflammation. Mobilization and stretching exercises should be initiated early to maintain shoulder mobility. The specific pathology will dictate the type of stretching to be performed. The goals of the stretching program are to reduce both inflammation and any capsular contractions present. In the initial stages of rehabilitation, avoid aggressive stretching. Stretching in external rotation and abduction should be avoided by throwers with suspected anterior instability. Strengthening exercises can be initiated as soon as the range of motion allows.

Phase Two: Bridging Flexibility to Strength

The strengthening program should be used to improve the dynamic stabilizers surrounding the shoulder girdle. Dynamic strengthening should develop not only strength but muscle power, endurance, and neuromuscular control. Strengthening exercises should begin at the base of the kinetic chain and work distal. Therefore, you should place emphasis on the scapular stabilizers. Key scapular strength-

ening exercises include scaption, shoulder protraction, and rowing. Progress can be monitored either by manual muscle testing or by measuring the lateral scapular glide distance. Bilateral comparison of the measurement between the inferior angle of the scapula and corresponding spinous process on the horizontal should be equal. With scapular stabilizer weakness, a deficit will exist. As scapular stability is increased, the difference in measurements will be reduced. The difference must be less than 1 centimeter before you can initiate functional progression. As the scapular stabilizers strengthen, attention can turn to the rotator cuff.

Phase Three: Advanced Strengthening

Your emphasis throughout the dynamic strengthening program should center on the performance of high-repetition and low-resistance exercises. Both concentric and eccentric muscle contractions should be used. Despite all the technical testing equipment available for rehabilitation, testing results should not be your definitive criteria for allowing an athlete to return to sport. There is a substantial difference in both the speed and specific movement performed on the testing devices compared to those used in actual throwing. Most equipment utilized for training and testing is confined to one of three cardinal planes and limited to one joint. This isolated pattern of movement is inconsistent with the throwing motion, which involves multiple movement patterns at both the shoulder and the elbow.

Testing equipment is not only inadequate in reproducing the throwing motion but is also unable to recreate the actual speeds of movement during throwing. Maximum angular velocities during the throwing motion approach 7000 degrees a second for shoulder internal rotation and 2000 degrees a second for elbow extension. These speeds are significantly greater than those which can be created on exercise equipment. So, for optimal rehabilitation, a specific functional throwing progression is required. For rehabilitation to be complete, the exact motion patterns and loads should gradually be reproduced—which leads us to the last stage of rehabilitation.

Phase Four: Return to Activity

The last phase of the rehabilitation program is the interval throwing program with a progressive return to play. This phase stresses the sport-specific action of the upper quarter. Once the athlete has been cleared for return to play, a program of short-distance tossing is progressed to longer throws with increased velocity. The gradual interval throwing program is set up to minimize risk for reinjury. Emphasize proper throwing mechanics.

Due to the difference between individuals and different pathologies, there is no set timetable for return-to-sport progressions. To reduce risk for reinjury, each program must be tailored to the needs of the individual athlete. Each stage of the interval program must be completed without complication or pain. In fact, pain should be your guideline for progression. It's not unusual for athletes to experience postexercise soreness, but sharp pain is an indicator to halt progression and reevaluate before continuing.

Interval throwing progressions have been developed by various clinicians. Figure 8.1 illustrates a typical progression as developed by Kevin Wilk. With a basic program established, variations for specific activities can be devised (see Figures 8.2-8.6, pp. 96-100).

◆ Simulated Game Situations

The last stage of functional progression for the throwing motion is completion of a simulated game situation. This is an attempt to evaluate the function of the throwing arm based on similar profiles. If the main goal of rehabilitation is the complete and painfree return of the athlete to previous level of function, you must use profile comparisons.

Using a simulated game/match situation allows you to employ the SAID principle. Defining the specific tasks that the athlete will be exposed to allows for the creation of a performance profile that will aid you in assessing functional strength, power, and endurance. In regard to the throwing athlete, the profile should include information about the number of pitches thrown per inning, the average number of innings pitched per game, the rest period between innings, and the percentages of different types of pitches thrown. Pitch selection is evaluated because with a still-present injury, a pitcher tends to throw more off-speed or breaking pitches to compensate for the inability to generate fastball velocity.

In one excellent study (Coleman, Axe, & Andrews, 1987), information was gathered on ma-

jor league pitchers and a profile thereby generated. Functional strength was reflected in the velocity of the fastball. The mile-per-hour change in fastball velocity per innings pitched was regarded as a function of the athlete's ability to maintain power or endurance. Pitching accuracy was evaluated by the fastball-for-strike ratio.

Results of the Coleman study (Coleman, Axe, & Andrews, 1987) indicate that the typical starting pitcher in the major league pitches 6-1/3 innings per game. Approximately 15% of his starts result in completion of the full 9 innings. The average number of pitches per inning was 15, and the most frequent pitch was the fastball (55.7%). The average fastball velocity in the first inning pitched was 87 miles per hour. The decrease in velocity per inning was calculated at 2% per inning. The fastball-for-strike ratio was approximately 64%. The rest period between innings was 9 minutes.

Based on this functional profile, a simulated game situation using the SAID principle can be created. The simulated game should follow a 15-minute warm-up period in which 50 to 80 pitches are thrown progressively faster. Duration should be 5 to 8 innings with 12 to 18 pitches each. The pitch selection should include 6 to 10 fastballs each inning. The rest interval between innings should be about 9 minutes.

The most important consideration in the simulated game situation is the assessment of throwing endurance. The ability to maintain velocity through a given inning is critical to a pitcher's success. The athlete is allowed a full return to sport if she or he shows a decrease of less than 1 to 1.5 miles per hour during the first 5 to 6 innings and has a good fastball-for-strike ratio. Additionally, throwing velocity must be within 3 miles per hour of preinjury average with no pain present during throwing. We recommend that the number of days between simulated games and the number of simulated games pitched before return to sport be based on each specific team's standards.

◆ Summary

As we've seen in this chapter, the complicated neuromuscular control needed for throwing cannot be left to chance in the traditional rehabilitation setting. A graduated functional progression for return to throwing is critical to success in the rehabilitation program.

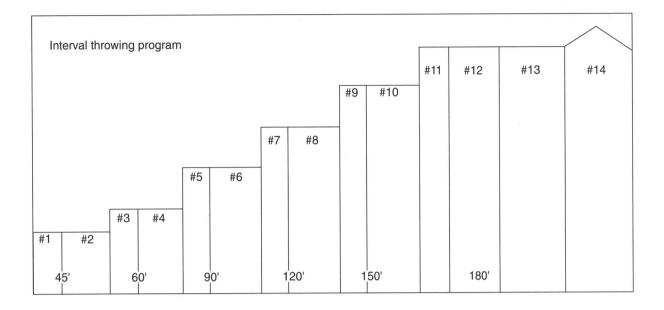

45' Phase

Step 1: A) Warm-up throwing
B) 45' (25 throws)
C) Rest 15 minutes
D) Warm-up throwing
E) 45' (25 throws)

Step 2: A) Warm-up throwing
B) 45' (25 throws)
C) Rest 10 minutes
D) Warm-up throwing
E) 45' (25 throws)
F) Rest 10 minutes
G) Warm-up throwing
H) 45' (25 throws)

60' Phase

Step 3: A) Warm-up throwing
B) 60' (25 throws)
C) Rest 15 minutes
D) Warm-up throwing
E) 60' (25 throws)

Step 4: A) Warm-up throwing
B) 60' (25 throws)
C) Rest 10 minutes
D) Warm-up throwing
E) 60' (25 throws)
F) Rest 10 minutes
G) Warm-up throwing
H) 60' (25 throws)

90' Phase

Step 5: A) Warm-up throwing
B) 90' (25 throws)
C) Rest 15 minutes

D) Warm-up throwing
E) 90' (25 throws)

Step 6: A) Warm-up throwing
B) 90' (25 throws)
C) Rest 10 minutes
D) Warm-up throwing
E) 90' (25 throws)
F) Rest 10 minutes
G) Warm-up throwing
H) 90' (25 throws)

120' Phase

Step 7: A) Warm-up throwing
B) 120' (25 throws)
C) Rest 15 minutes
D) Warm-up throwing
E) 120' (25 throws)

Step 8: A) Warm-up throwing
B) 120' (25 throws)
C) Rest 10 minutes
D) Warm-up throwing
E) 120' (25 throws)
F) Rest 10 minutes
G) Warm-up throwing
H) 120' (25 throws)

150' Phase

Step 9: A) Warm-up throwing
B) 150' (25 throws)
C) Rest 15 minutes
D) Warm-up throwing
E) 150' (25 throws)

Step 10: A) Warm-up throwing

B) 150' (25 throws)
C) Rest 10 minutes
D) Warm-up throwing
E) 150' (25 throws)
F) Rest 10 minutes
G) Warm-up throwing
H) 150' (25 throws)

180' Phase

Step 11: A) Warm-up throwing
B) 180' (25 throws)
C) Rest 15 minutes
D) Warm-up throwing
E) 180' (25 throws)

Step 12: A) Warm-up throwing
B) 180' (25 throws)
C) Rest 10 minutes
D) Warm-up throwing
E) 180' (25 throws)
F) Rest 10 minutes
G) Warm-up throwing
H) 180' (25 throws)

Step 13: A) Warm-up throwing
B) 180' (25 throws)
C) Rest 10 minutes
D) Warm-up throwing
E) 180' (25 throws)
F) Rest 10 minutes
G) Warm-up throwing
H) 180' (50 throws)

Step 14: Begin throwing off the mound or return to respective position.

Figure 8.1 An interval throwing program.

From: Kevin Wilk, PT, Director of Sports Medicine, Healthsouth Rehab—Birmingham, AL.

Interval Throwing Program Starting off the Mound

Stage One: Fastball only

Step 1:	Interval throwing	(Use interval throwing to 120' phase as warm-up)
	15 throws off mound, 50%	
Step 2:	Interval throwing	
	30 throws off mound, 50%	
Step 3:	Interval throwing	
	45 throws off mound, 50%	
Step 4:	Interval throwing	All throwing off the mound should be done in the
	60 throws off mound, 50%	presence of your pitching coach to stress proper
Step 5:	Interval throwing	throwing mechanics
	30 throws off mound, 75%	
Step 6:	30 throws off mound, 75%	
	45 throws off mound, 50%	
Step 7:	45 throws off mound, 75%	
	15 throws off mound, 50%	
Step 8:	60 throws off mound, 75%	

Stage Two: Fastball only

Step 9:   45 throws off mound, 75%
            15 throws in batting practice
Step 10:   45 throws off mound, 75%
            30 throws in batting practice
Step 11:   45 throws off mound, 75%
            45 throws in batting practice

Stage Three

Step 11:   30 throws off mound, 75% warm-up
            15 throws off mound, 50% breaking balls
            45-60 throws on batting practice (fastball only)
Step 12:   30 throws off mound, 75%
            30 breaking balls, 75%
            30 throws in batting practice
Step 13   30 throws off mound, 75%
            60 to 90 throws in batting practice, 25% breaking balls

---

Figure 8.2   Return to pitching program (off the mound).

From: Kevin Wilk, PT, Director of Sports Medicine, Healthsouth Rehab—Birmingham, AL.

Interval Golf Rehab Program

1st week

Monday	*Tuesday*	*Wednesday*
5 min. chip and putt	5 min chip and putt	5 min. chip and putt
5 min. rest	5 min. rest	5 min. rest
5 min. chip	5 min. chip	5 min. chip
	5 min. rest	5 min. rest
	5 min. chip	5 min. chip

2nd week

10 min. chip	10 min. chip	10 min. short iron
10 min. rest	10 min. rest	10 min. rest
10 min. short iron	10 min. short iron	10 min. short iron
	10 min. rest	10 min. rest
	10 min. short iron	10 min. short iron

3rd week

10 min. short iron	10 min. short iron	10 min. short iron
10 min. rest	10 min. rest	10 min. rest
10 min. long iron	10 min. long iron	10 min. long iron
10 min. rest	10 min. rest	10 min. rest
10 min. long iron	10 min. long iron	10 min. long iron

4th week

Repeat last Tuesday	Play 9 holes	Play 18 holes

Flexibility exercises before hitting.
Use ice after hitting.

Figure 8.3   Return to golf progression.

From: Kevin Wilk, PT, Director of Sports Medicine, Healthsouth Rehab—Birmingham, AL.

Medial Tennis Elbow Practice Schedule

Progress if no pain increase

Advanced elite player		Recreational player	
Day 1	15 min. — B only (two-handed) (no late strokes)	Day 1	15 min. —L only
Day 2	20 min. — B (two-handed) L few F (two-handed)	Day 2	20 min. — L;B
Day 3	30 min. — B;L; Few F (no T)	Day 3	30 min. — L;B;F (no late strokes) (no topspin ever)
Day 4	35 min. — B;L;BV;F (no T)	Day 4	40 min. — L;B;F;BV;
Day 5	40 min. —B;L;BV;F (no T) few O (to front court only)	Day 5	45 min. — L;B;F;BV; few O
Day 6	45 min. — B;L;BV;F (no T) O (to front court only)	Day 6	1 hr. — L;B;F;BV; O
Day 7	1 hr. — same as day 6	Day 7	1 hr. — L;B;BV;F;O; few S
Day 8	1 hr. — B;L;BV;F;FV (no T) FV (no late strokes ever)	Day 8	1 hr. — L;B;F;BV;O;S;F (no late strokes ever)
Day 9	1 hr. — B;L;BV;F (no T) O;FV few S (no AT)	Day 9	Resume normal practice play schedule
Day 10	1 hr. (AM) as day 9 15 min. (PM) B;L;F		
Day 11	1 hr. (AM) B;L;BV;F;(no T) O;FV;S (no T or AT) 30 min. (PM) B;L;BV;F; (no T)		
Day 12	1 hr. (AM) B;L;BV;F;O;FV;S (no T or AT) 45 min. (PM) B;L;BV;F;O		
Day 13	1 hr. (AM) same as day 12 1 hr. (PM) same as AM		
Day 14	1 hr. (AM) B;L;BV;F 1 hr. (PM) as AM		

F = forehand	B = backhand	S = serve	
FV = forward volley	BV= backhand volley	SL = slice	
U = underspin	T = topspin	AT = American twist	
FL = flat	O = overhead	FL = forehand lob	
BL = backhand lob	L = lob (either F or B)		

Progression rules

1. Day progression refers to actual playing day, not chronological
2. Gradual progression is the key to success.
3. It is important to keep eye on the ball. No late strokes.
4. Ice sore elbow immediately after play.

Figure 8.4   Return to tennis program following medial epicondylitis.

Adapted from Nirsch/PR Arm Care, 1981.

Lateral Tennis Elbow Practice Schedule

Progress if no pain increase

Advanced elite player			Recreational player		
Day 1	15 min.	— F only	Day 1	15 min.	—F only
Day 2	20 min.	— F;FL; few F	Day 2	30 min.	— F;FL; few FV
Day 3	30 min.	— F;FL;FV; few O (to F court only)	Day 3	30 min.	— F;FL;FV; few O
Day 4	35 min.	— F;FL;FV;O; few S	Day 4	45 min.	— F;FL;FV;O
Day 5	40 min.	— F;FL;FV;O;S (no SL;T; or AT)	Day 5	1 hr.	— F;FL;O;S; few B (two-handed)
Day 6	45 min.	— as day 5	Day 6	1 hr.	— F;FV;FL;O;S;BV (two-handed) B
Day 7	1 hr.	— as day 6	Day 7	1 hr.	— F;FV;L;O;S;B;BF (two-handed) B
Day 8	1 hr.	— F;FL;FV;O;S; (no SL or AT) few B (two-handed)	Day 8	1 hr.	— F;FV;L;O;S;B

Advanced elite player		
Day 9	1 hr.	— F;FL;FV;O;S;B (no AT) (no BV)
Day 10	1 hr.	— F;FV;L;O;S; (no AT) B (no U)
Day 11	1 hr.	(AM) as day 10
	20 min.	(PM) as day 10
Day 12	1 hr.	(AM) as day 11
	45 min.	(PM) F;FV;L;O
Day 13	1 hr.	(AM) F;FV;L;O;S;F; few BV (no U)
	45 min.	(PM) F;FV;L;O;S
Day 14	1 hr.	(AM) F;FV;L;O;S;B;BV
	1 hr.	(PM) as AM
Day 15		Resume normal practice play schedule

Recreational player:

Day 9   Resume normal practice play schedule
Day progression refers to actual playing days, not chronological days.

F = forehand	B = backhand	S = serve
FV = forward volley	BV = backhand volley	SL = slice
U = underspin	T = topspin	AT = American twist
FL = flat	O = overhead	FL = forehand lob
BL = backhand lob	L = lob (either F or B)	

Progression rules

1. Gradual progression is the key to success.
2. Keep eye on ball. No late strokes.
3. Two-handed backhand is more protective of the elbow.
4. Ice sore elbow immediately after play.

Figure 8.5   Return to tennis program following lateral epicondylitis.

Adapted from Nirsch/PR Arm Care, 1981.

Tennis Shoulder Practice Schedule

Progress if no pain increase

Advanced elite player			Recreational player		
Day 1	30 min.	— F;FV;L	Day 1	30 min.	—F;FV;L
Day 2	45 min.	— as day 1	Day 2	45 min.	— as day 1
Day 3	45 min.	— F;FV;L;B	Day 3	1 hr.	— as day 1
		(low—waist high or below)			
Day 4	45 min.	— as day 3	Day 4	1 hr.	— F;FV;L;B
Day 5	1 hr.	— F;FV;L;F; few BV	Day 5	1 hr.	— F;FV;L;BV
		(low—waist high or below)			
Day 6	1 hr.	— F;FV;L;B;BV (low)	Day 6	1 hr.	— as day 5
Day 7	1 hr.	— as day 6	Day 7	1 hr.	— F;FV;L;B;BV; few O (easy)
Day 8	1 hr.	(AM) as day 7	Day 8	1 hr.	— as day 7
	30 min.	(PM) F;FV;L;B;BV (low)			
Day 9	1 hr.	(AM) F;FV;L;B	Day 9	1 hr.	— F;FV;L;B;BV;O;S (easy)
Day 10	1 hr.	(AM) F;FV;L;B;O (easy) few S (easy)	Day 10	1 hr.	— as day 9
	1 hr.	(PM) as in AM			
Day 11	1 hr.	(AM)F;FV;L;B;BV;O (easy) S (easy)	Day 11	1 hr.	— F;FV;L;B;BV;O;S
	1 hr.	(PM) as in AM			
Day 12	1 hr.	(AM) F;FV;L;B;BV;O;S (easy)	Day 12	Return to normal practice-play schedule.	
	1 hr.	(PM)as in AM			
Day 13	1 hr.	(AM) F;FV;L;B;BV;O;S			
	1 hr.	(PM) as in AM			
Day 14		as day 13			
Day 15		Resume normal practice-play schedule			

F	= forehand	B	= backhand	S	= serve
FV	= forward volley	BV	= backhand volley	SL	= slice
U	= underspin	T	= topspin	AT	= American twist
FL	= flat	O	= overhead	FL	= forehand lob
BL	= backhand lob	L	= lob (either F or B)		

Progression rules

1. Day progression refers to actual playing day, not chronological days.
2. Gradual progression in the key to success.
3. It is important to keep eye on the ball. No late strokes.
4. Ice sore elbow immediately after play.

Figure 8.6   Return to tennis program following shoulder injury.

Adapted from Nirsch/PR Arm Care, 1981.

Glossary

Ankle strategy—a balance mechanism to bring the body's center of gravity within the base of support by moving the body as a relatively rigid mass about fixed ankle joints through muscular contractions proceeding in a distal to proximal direction.

Arm hopping—an upper extremity unilateral support drill in which the athlete runs to a predetermined point, places the involved arm on the ground, absorbs the body weight through the arm, then pushes off the arm back into a running position and repeats the sequence at predetermined intervals.

Arm spin—an upper extremity unilateral support drill performed in a modified push-up position. The athlete uses the weight-bearing arm as a pivot point to spin in circles in clockwise and counterclockwise directions.

Bilateral support activities—upper or lower extremity activities in which both arms or both legs are fixed in a weight-bearing position.

Carriage—a component of the successful completion of a functional progression task in which the athlete demonstrates symmetry in weight shift, weight acceptance, and fluid movement patterns.

Co-contraction test—a functional test designed to dynamically assess knee stability after injury to the anterior cruciate ligament. The athlete performs lateral movements in a semicircle against the resistance of elastic cords.

Collision sport—a sport in which direct physical contact with an opposing player is allowed by the rules. Examples are hockey, lacrosse, and American football.

Combat sport—a sport in which the prime objective is to exert control over one's opponent by physical means. Examples are wrestling, boxing, judo, and other martial arts.

Confidence—a component of the successful completion of a functional progression task in which the athlete competently performs a given skill with physical ease and psychological self-assuredness.

Contact sport—a sport in which physical contact does occur but is not commonly allowed by the rules. Examples are basketball, baseball, and softball.

Control—a component of the successful completion of a functional progression task in which the athlete demonstrates automatic, unrestricted, efficient performance of a desired skill.

Countermovements—movements usually performed in combat sports in which the athlete attempts to negate the effectiveness of the opponent's controlling maneuvers.

Counterpunch—a force-delivery maneuver in combat sports in which the athlete attempts to strike the opponent at the same time the opponent is delivering a striking blow.

Crossover cut—an acceleration/deceleration drill in which the athlete decelerates, plants the involved leg, brings the uninvolved leg in front of the pivot leg, and accelerates at a 90° angle in the same direction of the involved leg.

Damped jump—a repetitive jumping activity in which the eccentric muscle contraction involved with landing from the jump is characterized by excessive knee flexion, allowing a slow transition to the following jump and decreased height of the subsequent jump.

Davis's Law—an important principle governing the functional progression program. The law states that injured soft tissue heals according to the stress placed on it during healing.

Depth jump—an advanced plyometric drill in which the athlete stands on an object of a predetermined height and steps off the object. As both feet land on the floor, the athlete immediately jumps as far forward or as high as possible.

Down-position activities—functional progression activities in combat sports in which both participants perform from other than the standing position (usually from the quadruped, kneeling, or prone positions).

Dynamic movement testing—plyometric vertical or horizontal jumping or hopping used as a functional test.

Dynamic restraints—structures that maintain normal joint stability through muscular contraction, namely muscle or tendon.

Escape—a maneuver in combat sports in which the athlete completely removes himself from the physical control of an opponent.

Extrafusal muscle fibers—skeletal muscle fibers directly responsible for muscular contraction.

Figure-eight drill—an acceleration/deceleration drill in which the athlete changes direction of movement in connected circular patterns that resemble the numeral 8.

Force acceptance—functional progression activities in which the individual receives physical contact. Examples are being tackled, being checked, or blocking a karate kick.

Force delivery—functional progression activities in which the athlete imparts physical contact to an opponent. Examples are tackling, checking in hockey, or a karate kick.

Functional progression—a series of sport-specific movement patterns progressed according to the physical and psychological tolerance of an individual to prepare the individual to return to preinjury sport function.

Functional testing—maximal performance of an activity to assess an individual's performance of that specific activity.

Functional training—performance of repetitive activities to improve an athlete's performance of that specific activity.

Golgi ligament endings—a slowly adapting articular mechanoreceptor sensitive to changes in tension within a ligament.

Golgi-Mazzoni corpuscles—a slowly adapting articular mechanoreceptor sensitive to perpendicular compression of the joint.

Golgi tendon organ—a deep, muscle-tendon mechanoreceptor responsible for monitoring tension within the muscle-tendon unit.

Hip strategy—a balance mechanism that brings the body's center of gravity within the base of support through a quick response centered about the hips, with muscular contractions proceeding in a proximal to distal direction.

Intrafusal muscle fibers—the muscle fibers containing the tension monitoring and tension regulating muscle spindle.

Inverted push-up—a bilateral support, upper extremity drill in which the individual performs a traditional push-up without assistance from the lower extremities.

Limits of stability—the outermost range in any direction a person can lean from the vertical without altering the base of support.

Loaded activities—any functional progression activity in which resistance is applied to the individual, whether in the form of weights or the body weight of an opponent.

Mechanoreceptor—specialized groups of cells that function to convert mechanical distortion of tissue into electrical activity that is subsequently transmitted into the central nervous system.

Microtrauma—injury produced by submaximal loading of a body part that occurs in a repetitive, cyclic fashion.

Mini-squat—a bilateral support lower extremity activity in which the individual performs a squat until the thighs are parallel with the ground, while maintaining the lower legs perpendicular to the ground.

Motor control—the integration of sensory information from the body through the central nervous system that yields coordinated volitional movement.

Multiplane drills—activities performed in a combination of front-to-back and side-to-side directions.

Muscle spindle—a complex receptor located within intrafusal muscle fiber that is responsible for monitoring the tension within the muscle-tendon unit.

Nociceptors—free nerve ending mechanoreceptors.

Open kinetic chain—movement of the lower or upper extremity in which the distal segment of the limb is free to move. Examples of open chain motion are seated knee extensions or bicep curls.

Pacinian corpuscles—a rapidly adapting articular mechanoreceptor responsible for sensing the initiation and/or cessation of joint movement.

Plyometrics—a mode of training developed in Eastern Europe that emphasizes a quick eccentric muscle contraction to produce a greater subsequent concentric muscle contraction.

Proprioception—a specialized sense of touch referring to all the neural input originating from the muscles, tendons, ligaments, and capsule surrounding a joint.

Recovery time—rest between sets of exercise.

Ruffini endings—a slowly adapting articular mechanoreceptor responsible for sensing stretch within the joint capsule (e.g., stretch produced by changes in intracapsular fluid).

SAID principle—Specific Adaptations to Imposed Demands. An important principle governing the functional progression program. The principle states that for an athlete to safely return to sport after being injured, stresses placed on him or her during rehabilitation must specifically address the demands that he or she will assume upon return to preinjury activities.

SEMO drill—an acceleration/deceleration functional test that incorporates forward, backward, and diagonal running with right and left lateral shuffling.

Shuttle run—an acceleration/deceleration functional test that incorporates forward sprinting and quick changes of direction.

Sidestep cut—an acceleration/deceleration drill in which the athlete decelerates, plants the involved leg, and then accelerates at a 90° angle in the opposite direction of the planted leg.

Single-plane drills—activities performed in either in a front-to-back or side-to-side direction.

Sit-out—a countermovement in wrestling in which the athlete quickly moves from a quadruped position to a seated position on the mat.

Sprawl—a countermovement utilized in wrestling in which the athlete quickly moves from a quadruped position on the wrestling mat to a prone position.

Static restraints—noncontractile structures responsible for maintaining normal joint stability, namely joint capsule and ligaments found inside and/or outside of the joint.

Static testing—balance assessment activities performed in a stationary position.

Stepping strategy—a balance mechanism employed when the limits of stability are exceeded that requires the individual to move the feet to place the center of gravity within the new base of support.

Step-up—a lower extremity unilateral support functional test or functional progression drill in which hip and knee extension of the involved leg brings the individual up onto a step of a predetermined height.

T-drill—an acceleration/deceleration functional test involving forward sprinting combined with lateral shuffling or pivoting movements performed over an area resembling the letter T.

Transitional drills—functional progression or functional testing activities performed after the successful completion of upper or lower extremity bilateral support drills but prior to initiating unilateral support activities.

Undamped jump—a repetitive jumping activity in which the eccentric muscle contraction involved with landing from the jump is characterized by minimal knee flexion, a rapid transition to the following jump, and increased height of the subsequent jump.

Unilateral support activities—upper or lower extremity activities in which only one arm or one leg is fixed in a weight-bearing position.

Unloaded activities—any functional progression activity in which the body weight of the athlete is the only resistance encountered.

Up-position activities—activities in combat sport functional progression in which both individuals perform from standing positions.

Wheelbarrow drill—an upper extremity drill in which the athlete alternately accepts weight on each arm while the lower extremities are not allowed to make contact with the ground.

Wolf's Law—an important principle governing the functional progression program that states that injured bone heals according to the stress placed upon it during the healing process.

References

Adams, T. (1984). An investigation of selected plyometric training exercises on muscular leg strength and power. *Track and Field Quarterly Review*, **84**, 36-40.

Asmussen, E., & Bonde-Peterson, F. (1974). Storage of elastic energy in skeletal muscles in man. *Acta Physiologica Scandinavica*, **91**, 385.

Barber, S.D., Noyes, F.R., Mangine, R.E., McCloskey, J.W., & Hartman, W. (1990). Quantitative assessment of functional limitations in normal and anterior cruciate ligament-deficient knees. *Clinical Orthopedics*, **255**, 204-214.

Barrack, R.L., Bruckner, J.D., Kneisl, J., Inman, W.S., & Alexander, A.H. (1990). The outcome of nonoperatively treated complete tears of the anterior cruciate ligament in active young adults. *Clinical Orthopedics*, **259**, 192-199.

Baxendale, R.N., & Ferrell, W.R. (1980). Modulation of transmission in flexion reflex pathways by knee joint afferent discharge in the decerebrate cat. *Brain Research*, **202**, 497-500.

Baxendale, R.N., & Ferrell, W.R. (1982). The effect of elbow joint afferent discharge on transmission in forearm flexion reflex pathways to biceps and triceps brachii in decerebrate cats. *Brain Research*, **247**, 57-63.

Bielik, E., Chu, D., & Costello, F. (1986). Roundtable: Practical considerations for utilizing plyometrics. Part 1: *National Strength and Conditioning Association Journal*. **8**, 14.

Bloomfield, J., Fricker, P.A., & Fitch, K.D. (Eds.) (1992). *Textbook of science and medicine in sport*. Champaign, IL: Human Kinetics.

Bosco, C., & Komi, P.V. (1979). Potentiation of the mechanical behavior of the human skeletal muscle through prestretching. *Acta Physiologica Scandinavica*, **106**, 467.

Bosco, C., & Komi, P.V. (1982). Muscle elasticity in athletes. In *Exercise and sports biology* (pp. 109-117). P.V. Komi (Ed.). Champaign, IL: Human Kinetics.

Bosco, C., Tarkka, J., & Komi, P.V. (1982). Effect of elastic energy and myoelectric potentiation of triceps surea during stretch cycle exercise.

International Journal of Sports Medicine, **2**, 137.

Buckley, S.L., Barrack, R.L., & Alexander, A.H. (1989). The natural history of conservatively treated partial anterior cruciate ligament tears. *American Journal of Sports Medicine*, **17**, 221-225.

Burgess, P.R. (1982). Signal of kinesthetic information by peripheral sensory receptors. *Annual Review of Neuroscience*, **5**, 171.

Cafarelli, E., & Bigland, B. (1979). Sensation of static force in muscles of different length. *Experimental Neurology*, **65**, 511-525.

Chu, D. (1984). Plyometric exercise. *National Strength and Conditioning Association Journal*, **6**, 56.

Chu, D. (1989, December). *Conditioning/plyometrics*. Paper presented at Tenth Annual Sports Medicine Team Concept Meeting, San Francisco, CA.

Chu, D. (1992). *Jumping into plyometrics*. Champaign, IL: Leisure Press.

Chu, D., & Plumer, L. (1984). The language of plyometrics. *National Strength and Conditioning Association Journal*, **6**, 30.

Coleman, A.E., Axe, M.J., & Andrews, J.R. (1987). Performance profile-directed simulated game: An objective functional evaluation for baseball pitchers. *Journal of Orthopedic Sports Physical Therapy*, **9**, 101-105.

Cook, E.E., Gray, V.L., Savinar-Nogue, E., & Medeiros, R. (1987). Shoulder antagonistic strength ratios: A comparison between college-level baseball pitchers and nonpitchers. *Journal of Orthopedic Sports Physical Therapy*, **8**, 451-461.

Cross, M.J., Gibbs, N.J., & Bryant, G.J. (1989). An analysis of the sidestep cutting manoeuvre. *American Journal of Sports Medicine*, **17**, 363-366.

Cross, M.M., & McCloskey, D.L. (1973). Position sense following surgical removal of joints in man. *Brain*, **55**, 443-445.

de Andrade, J.R., Grant, C., & Dixon, A.J. (1965). Joint distension and reflex muscle inhibition in the knee. *Journal of Bone Joint Surgery*, **47**, 412-422.

Dillman, C.J. (1991, January). *Biomechanics of pitching*. Paper presented at the Injuries in Baseball Conference, Birmingham, AL.

Doss, W.S., & Karpovich, P.V. (1965). A comparison of concentric, eccentric, and isometric strength of elbow flexors. *Journal of Applied Physiology*, **20**, 351-353.

Dunsenev, C.I. (1979). Strength training for jumpers. *Soviet Sports Review*, **14**, 2.

Dunsenev, C.I. (1982). Strength training for jumpers. *Track and Field Quarterly Review*, **82**, 4.

Ekholm, J., Ekland, G., & Skoglund, S. (1960). On the reflex effects from the knee joint of the cat. *Acta Physiologica Scandinavica*, **50**, 167-174.

Eklund, J. (1972). Position sense and state of contraction: the effects of vibration. *Journal of Neurological and Neurosurgical Psychiatry*, **35**, 606.

Elmqvist, L.G., Lorentzon, R., Langstrom, M., & Fugl-Meyer, A.R. (1988). Reconstruction of the anterior cruciate ligament: Long-term effects of different knee angles at primary immobilization and different modes of early training. *American Journal of Sports Medicine*, **16**, 455-462.

Freeman, M., & Wyke, B. (1967a). The innervation of the knee joint: Anatomical and historical study in the cat. *Journal of Anatomy*, **101**, 505-532.

Freeman, M., & Wyke, B. (1967b). Articular reflexes at the ankle joint: An electromyographic study of normal and abnormal influences of ankle joint mechanoreceptors upon reflex activity in the leg muscles. *British Journal of Surgery*, **54**, 990-1001.

Friden, T., Zatterstrom, R., Lindstrand, A., & Moritz, U. (1990). Disability in anterior cruciate ligament insufficiency: An analysis of 19 untreated patients. *Acta Orthopaedica Scandinavica*, **61**, 131-135.

Gandevia, S.C., & McCloskey, D.I. (1976). Joint sense, muscle sense, and their combination as position sense, measured at the distal interphalangeal joint of the middle finger. *Journal of Physiology*, **260**, 387-407.

Gauffin, H., Pettersson, Y., Tegner, Y., & Tropp, H. (1990). Function testing in patients with old rupture of the anterior cruciate ligament. *International Journal of Sports Medicine*, **11**, 73-77.

Gauffin, H., Pettersson, G., & Tropp, H. (1990). Kinematic analysis of one-leg long hopping in patients with an old rupture of the anterior cruciate ligament. *Clinical Biomechanics*, **5**, 41-46.

Glencross, D., & Thornton, E. (1981). Position sense following joint injury. *Journal of Sports Medicine Physical Fitness*, **21**, 23.

Goodwin, G.M., McCloskey, D.I., & Matthews, P.C. (1972). The contribution of muscle afferents to kinesthesia shown by vibration induced illusions of movement and by effects of paralyzing joint afferents. *Brain*, **95**, 705-748.

Gould, J., & Davies, G. (Eds.) (1985). *Orthopaedic and sports physical therapy*. St Louis: C.V. Mosby.

Gray, G. (1986). Rehabilitation of running injuries: Biomechanical and proprioceptive considerations. *Topics in Acute Care and Trauma Rehabilitation*. Gaithersburg, MD: Aspen Publishers.

Gray, G. (1990). *Chain reaction: Successful strategies for closed chain testing and rehabilitation*. Adrian, MI: Wynn Marketing.

Griggs, P., Finerman, G.A., & Riley L.H. (1973). Joint position sense after total hip replacement. *Journal of Bone Joint Surgery*, **55**, 1016-1025.

Haddad, B. (1953). Protection of afferent fibers from the knee joint to the cerebellum of the cat. *American Journal of Physiology*, **172**, 511-514.

Harter, R.A., Osternig, L.R., Singer, K.M., James, S.L., Larson, R.L., & Jones, D.C. (1988). Long-term evaluation of knee stability and function following surgical reconstruction for anterior cruciate ligament insufficiency. *American Journal of Sports Medicine*, **16**, 434-443.

Hellenbrandt, F.A. (1978). Motor learning reconsidered: A study of change. In *Neurophysiologic Approaches to Therapeutic Exercise*. Philadelphia: F.A. Davis.

Henning, C.E., Lynch, M.A., & Glick, K.R. (1985). An in vivo strain gauge study of elongation of the anterior cruciate ligament. *American Journal of Sports Medicine*, **13**, 22-26.

Horack, F.B., & Washer, L.M. (1986). Central programming of postural movements: Adaptation to altered support surface configurations. *Journal of Neurophysiology*, **55**, 1369-1381.

Indelicato, P.A., Hermansdorfer, J., & Huegel, M. (1990). Nonoperative management of complete tears of the medial collateral ligament of the knee in intercollegiate football players. *Clinical Orthopedics*, **256**, 174-177.

Jackson, D.W., Ashley, R.L., & Powell, J.W. (1974). Ankle sprains in young athletes: Relation of severity and disability. *Clinical Orthopedics*, **101**, 201-215.

Javorek, I. (1989). Plyometrics. *National Strength and Conditioning Association Journal*, **11**, 52.

Jensen, C. (1975). Pertinent facts about warming. *Athletic Journal*, **56**, 72.

Jokl, P., Kaplan, N., Stovell, P., & Keggi, K. (1987). Non-operative treatment of severe injuries to the medial and anterior cruciate ligaments of the knee. *Journal of Bone Joint Surgery*, **66A**, 741-744.

Katchajov, S., Gomgeraze, K., & Revson, A. (1976). Rebound jumps. *Modern Athlete and Coach*, **14**, 23.

Kegerreis, S. (1983). The construction and implementation of functional progression as a component of athletic rehabilitation. *Journal of Orthopedic Sports Physical Therapy*, **5**, 14-19.

Kegerreis, S., Malone, T., & McCarroll, J. (1984). Functional progressions: An aid to athletic rehabilitation. *Physical Sports Medicine*, **12**, 67-71.

Kegerreis, S., & Wetherald, T. (1987). The utilization of functional progressions in the rehabilitation of injured wrestlers. *Athletic Training*, **22**, 32-35.

Kennedy, J.C., Alexander, I.J., & Hayes, K.C. (1982). Nerve supply of the human knee and its functional importance. *American Journal of Sports Medicine*, **10**, 329-335.

Kirby, R.F. (1971). A simple test of agility. *Coach and Athlete*, **6**, 30-31.

Komi, P.V. (1984). Physiological and biomechanical correlates of muscle function: Effects of muscle structure and stretch-shortening cycle on force and speed. In Terjung (Ed.) *Exercise and Sports Sciences Review*. Lexington, KY: Collamore Press.

Lephart, S.M., Perrin, D.H., Fu, F.H., & Minger, K. (1991). Functional performance tests for the anterior cruciate ligament insufficient athlete. *Athletic Training*, **26**, 44-50.

Lundon, P. (1985). A review of plyometric training. *National Strength and Conditioning Association Journal*, **7**, 69.

Magee, D.J. (1992). *Orthopedic physical assessment*. Philadelphia: W.B. Saunders.

Markolf, K.L., Bargar, W.L., Shoemaker, S.C. & Amstutz, H.C. (1981). The role of joint load in knee stability. *Journal of Bone Joint Surgery*, **63**, 570-585.

Matthews, P.C. (1982). Where does Sherrington's "muscular sense" originate? Muscles, joints, corollary discharges? *Annual Review of Neuroscience*, **5**, 189.

McCloskey, D.I. (1978). Kinesthetic sensibility. *Physiology Review*, **58**, 763-820.

McMahon, L.M., Burdett, R.G., & Whitney, S.L. (1992). Effects of muscle group and placement site on reliability of hand-held dynamometry strength measurements. *Journal of Orthopedic Sports Physical Therapy*, **15**, 236-241.

Miller, J. (1973). Joint afferent fibers responding to muscle stretch, vibration, and contraction. *Brain Research*, **63**, 380-383.

Nasher, L.W., & McCollum, G. (1985). The organization of human postural movements: a formal basis and experimental synthesis. *Behavioral and Brain Sciences*, **8**, 135-172.

Nideffer, R.M. (1983). The injured athlete: Psychological factors in treatment. *Orthopaedic Clinics of North America*, **14**, 373-385.

Noyes, F.R., Torvik, P.J., Hyde, W.B., DeLucas, J.L. (1974). Biomechanics of ligament failure: An analysis of immobilization, exercise, and reconditioning effects in primates. *Journal of Bone Joint Surgery*, **56A**, 1406-1418.

O'Conner, B. (1984). The mechanoreceptor innervation of the posterior attachments of the lateral meniscus of the dog knee joint. *Journal of Anatomy*, **138**, 1526.

Odensten, M., Lysholm, J., & Gillquist, J. (1985). The course of partial anterior cruciate ligament ruptures. *American Journal of Sports Medicine*, **13**, 183-186.

Palmer, I. (1958). Pathophysiology of the medial ligament of the knee joint of the cat. *Acta Chirurgica Scandinavica*, **115**, 312-318.

Phillips, C.G., Powell, T.S., & Wiesendanger, M. (1971). Protection from low threshold muscle afferents of hand and forearm area 3A of Babson's cortex. *Journal of Physiology*, **217**, 419-446.

Rasch, P.J., Grabiner, M.D., Gregor, R.J., & Garhammer, J. (1989). *Kinesiology and applied anatomy* (7th edition). Philadelphia: Lea & Febiger.

Rowinski, M.J. (1988). *The role of eccentric exercise*. Shirley, NY: Biodex Corp., Pro Clinics, Inc.

Rowinski, M.J. (1990). Afferent neurobiology of the joint. In *Orthopaedic and Sports Physical Therapy*. St Louis: CV Mosby.

Schmidt, R.A. (1988). *Motor control and learning*. Champaign, IL: Human Kinetics.

Schulte, M.J., & Happel, L.T. (1990). Joint innervation in injury. *Clinical Sports Medicine*, **9**, 511-517.

Sherrington, C.S. (1906). On the proprioceptive system, especially in its reflex aspects. *Brain*, **29**, 467.

Spencer, J.D., Hayes, K.C., & Alexander, I.J. (1984). Knee joint effusion and quadriceps inhibition in man. *Archives of Physical Medicine and Rehabilitation*, **65**, 171-177.

Stanish, W.D., Rubinovich, R.M., & Curwin, S. (1986). Eccentric exercise in chronic tendinitis. *Clinical Orthopedics*, **208**, 65-68.

Stauber, W.T. (1989). Eccentric action of muscles: Physiology, injury and adaptation. In *Exercise and Sports Sciences Reviews*, Vol. 17 (pp. 187-212), K.B. Pandolf (Ed.). Edinburgh: Churchill Livingstone.

Tegner, Y., Lysholm, J., Lysholm, M., & Gillquist, J. (1986). A performance test to monitor rehabilitation and evaluate anterior cruciate ligament injuries. *American Journal of Sports Medicine*, **14**, 156-159.

Tippett, S.R. (1990a). *Coaches guide to sport rehabilitation* (pp. 121-125). Champaign, IL: Human Kinetics.

Tippett, S.R. (1990b). Sports rehabilitation concepts (pp. 9-14). In Sanders (Ed.) *Sports Physical Therapy*. Norwalk, CT: Appleton and Lange.

Trundle, T.L. (1984). *Cybex isokinetic testing and rehabilitation*. Greenville, SC: Ex-Spo.

Turek, S.L. (1984). *Orthopaedics: Principles and their application* (pp. 1269-1406). Philadelphia: J.B. Lippincott.

Verhoshanski, Y. (1967). Are depth jumps useful? *Track and Field*, **12**, 9.

Verhoshanski, Y. (1969). Perspectives in the improvement of speed-strength preparation of jumpers. *Yesis Review of Soviet Physical Education and Sports*, **4**, 28-29.

Verhoshanski, Y., & Chornonson, G. (1967). Jump exercise in sprint training. *Track and Field Quarterly Review*, **9**, 1909.

Voight, M., & Draovitch, P. (1991). Plyometrics. In Albert (Ed.) *Eccentric muscle training in sports and orthopedics*. New York: Churchill Livingstone.

Von Arx, F. (1984). Power development in the high jump. *Track Technique*, **88**, 2818-2819.

Wadsworth, C.T., & Krishan, R. (1987). Interater reliability of manual muscle testing and hand-held dynametric muscle testing. *Physical Therapy*, **67**, 1342-1347.

Walmsley, R.P., & Szybbo, C. (1987). A comparative study of the torque generated by the shoulder internal and external rotator muscles in different positions and at varying speeds. *Journal of Orthopedic Sports Physical Therapy*, **9**, 217-227.

Weiss, C.B., Lundberg, M., Hamberg, H., DeHaven, K.E., & Gillquist, J. (1989). Non-operative treatment of meniscal tears. *Journal of Bone Joint Surgery*, **71A**, 811-822.

Wikholw, J.B., & Bohannon, R.W. (1991). Handheld dynamometer measurements: Tester strength makes a difference. *Journal of Orthopedic Sports Physical Therapy*, **13**, 191-198.

Willis, W.D., & Grossman, R.G. (1981). *Medical neurobiology* (3rd edition). St Louis: CV Mosby.

Wilt, F. (1975). Plyometrics—what it is and how it works. *Athletic Journal*, **55B**, 76.

Woo, S.L., & Buckwater, J.A. (1987). *Injury and repair of the musculoskeletal soft tissues*. Park Ridge, IL: American Academy of Orthopaedic Surgeons.

Wyatt, M.P., & Edwards, A.M. (1981). Comparison of quadriceps and hamstring torque values during isokinetic exercise. *Journal of Orthopedic Sports Physical Therapy*, **3**, 48-56.

Yamamoto, S.K., Hartman, C.W., Feagin, J.A., & Kimball, G. (1975). Functional rehabilitation of the knee: A preliminary study. *Journal of Sports Medicine*, **3**, 288-291.

Zimny, M.L. (1988). Mechanoreceptors in articular tissues. *American Journal of Anatomy*, **182**, 16-32.

Index

Page numbers in **boldface** refer to terms in the glossary.

A

Acceleration (in throwing), 92

Acceleration/deceleration pivoting drills, 15, 50-51

Activity loads, progression of, 8-9. *See also* Loaded activities

Adams, T., 81

Aerobic dancing, 73

Aerobic endurance, 8, 49, 63, 84-85

Afferent mechanoreceptor input, 23, 24, 25, 76

Agility drills
    and co-contraction test, 44, **101**
    difficulty shuttle run, 42-43, **103**
    SEMO drill, 43-44, **103**
    T-drill cut, 43, **103**
    T-drill shuffle, 43, **103**

Agonist:antagonist ratios, 7

Agonist muscle activity, 21, 25

Alexander, I.J., 22

Alpha motoneurons, 21, 76

Amortization phase (of muscle contraction), 76-77

Amstutz, H.C., 25

Anaerobic endurance, 8, 49, 63

Analgesics, 6

Ankle dorsiflexion, 11

Ankle injuries
    functional classification of ankle sprains, 32
    inversion ankle sprain, 4, 9
    use of ankle disc in, 23

Ankle strategy (for automatic postural correction), 27, **101**

Ankle taping or bracing, 10

Antagonist muscle activity, 21, 23, 25

Anterior-posterior (AP) limits of stability, 26

Anxiety. *See* Stress, psychological

Arm hopping and spins (drill), 57-58, **101**

Arm spins, 38, 57-58, **101**

Articular mechanoreceptors
    debate about, 22
    Golgi-like receptors, 21, 25
    nociceptors, 21, **102**
    Pacinian corpuscles, 20-21, 25, **102**
    Ruffini endings, 20, 25, **102-103**

Articularis cubiti muscle, 22

Articularis genu muscle, 22

Ashley, R.L., 32

Asmussen, E., 81

Assessment. *See* Functional testing

Athletes
    medical history of, 77
    pairing in drills, 52, 53, 64, 70, 71
    physical benefits of functional progression for, 4-5
    psychological benefits of functional progression for, 5-6

B

Balance. *See* Standing balance

Bargar, W.L., 25

Baseball, 47, 83

Basic program
    acceleration/decleration pivoting drills, 15, 50-51
    bilateral nonsupport drills (jumping), 13-15, 39-41
    bilateral support drills (mini-squats), 10-11, 33-34, 38-39, 53-55, **102**
    cutting maneuver drills, 17-18
    figure-eight drills, 15-17, 71, **102**
    unilateral nonsupport drills (hopping), 15, 29-30, 31, 39-41
    unilateral support drills (step-ups), 11-13, 29, 36-39, **103**

Basketball, 4, 47, 73, 83

Baxendale, R.N., 22

Bench hops, 73

Bench jumps and hops, 40

Bilateral nonsupport drills (jumping), 13-15, 39-41

Bilateral support activities
  definition of, **101**
  drills (mini-squats), 10-11, 33-34, 38-39, 53-55, **102**
  tests, 33-36
Biodex Upper Body Cycle, 84
Blocking, 65
Blocking and tackling dummies, stationary and hand-held, 51, 59, 65
Blocking sleds, 51, 59
Body position and movement
  and balance, 25-27, 63
  cognitive awareness of, 23-24
Body sway
  and automatic postural responses, 27
  and balance, 26
  degree of (sway envelope), 26
  measure of, 25
Bonde-Peterson, F., 81
Borzov, Valery, 73
Bosco, C., 75, 77, 81
Bounding, 79
Boxing, 64
Braces, 23

C
Carriage, 9, 10, **101**
Center of gravity, 25-27
Central nervous system (CNS), 19. *See also* Neurophysiology
Chornonson, G., 80
Chu, D., 78, 79
Circuit training, 80
Closed kinetic-chain rehabilitation exercise, 24-25, 32, 77-78
Co-contraction test, 44, **101**
Coleman, A.E., 94
Collision sports
  definition of, 47, **101**
  injuries in, 47
Combat drills, 64
Combat sports
  definition of, 63, **101**
  injuries in, 63
Competition in combat sports, 64
Compression, intermittent or constant, 6, 10
Confidence. *See* Self-confidence
Contact punching, 67
Contact sports
  definition of, 47, **101**

injuries in, 47
Contraction of muscles, 21, 22, 23, 74-76
Contralateral plantar flexors, functional testing of, 37-38
Control, 9, 10, **101**
Countermovement
  definition of, **101**
  drills for, 69
Counterpunching, 66, 67, **101**
Crawling drill, 54-55
Crossover cut, 17, **101**
Cross-training, 85
Cryotherapy, 6, 10
Cutting drills
  cutting maneuver drills, 17-18
  figure-eight drills, 15-17, 71, **102**
  following lower extremity injury, 50
  T-drill cut, 43
Cutting maneuver drills, 17-18

D
Damped jumps, 75, **101**
Davis's Law, 4, 6, **101**
de Andrade, J.R., 22
Deconditioning, 84
Deep muscle-tendon related receptors
  Golgi tendon organs (GTOs), 21-22, 76, 77, **102**
  muscle spindle, 21, 23, 24, 76, **102**
Depth jumping, 80-81, **101**
Diagonal jumping, 13
Difficulty shuttle run (drill), 42-43, **103**
Distance
  jumping and hopping for, 40-41
  progression of, 8, 52, 53, 85-87
Distance running, 83, 84-87
Dixon, A.J., 22
Down-position (on the mat) drills, 67, 68-69, **101**
Drez, Dr. David, 78
Duration of drills, 11, 52, 64, 66, 85-87
Dykes, 22
Dynamic movement testing, 78-79, **101**
Dynamic restraints, **101**

E
Eccentric control, functional testing of, 37
Ekholm, J., 22
Ekland, G., 22
Electrotherapeutic modalities, 6

Endurance, 8, 19, 49, 63, 84-85
Endurance training, 80
Equilibrium, 23, 25-27
Equipment, protective
    for collision and contact sports, 47, 51
    for combat sports, 63, 64, 65, 66, 70
Escape
    definition of, **102**
    drills for, 69
Evaluation. *See* Functional testing
Extrafusal muscle fibers, 21, **102**

F
Face-off position, 88
Fastex system, 41
Feagin, J.A., 3
Ferrell, W.R., 22
Figure-eight drills, 15-17, 71, **102**
Finerman, G.A., 24
Flexibility, 78, 93
Follow-through (in throwing), 92
Football, 47, 83
Footwork drills, 49
Force delivery and acceptance, single-plane and
        multiplane
    for collision and contact sports, 51-53, 59-61
    for combat sports, 64-71
    definition of, **102**
Force of muscles, 74-77
Form, proper, 64
Forward propulsion, 26
Forward rolls (drill), 58
4-point (modified push-up) position, 34-36, 38,
        53-54, **88**
Freeman, M., 22, 23
Free-style wrestling, 67
Frequency (of training), 79, 86, 87, 88
Front-to-back jumping, 13
Functional progression
    activity loads in, 8-9
    basic (sample) program for, 10-18
    benefits for the athlete, 4-6
    benefits for the rehabilitation professional, 6
    components of, 3-18
    definition of, 3, **102**
    distance progressions in, 8, 52, 53, 85-87
    drills for, 5, 10-18
    history of, 3-4
    implementation of program, 8-9

integration with formal rehabilitation, 9-10
    for nonstriking sports, 67-71
    physical benefits for athlete
        maximization of postinjury performance,
            4-5
        promotion of healing, 4, 6
    program assessment, 9
    program prerequisites, 6-8
    program progression, 8-9
    psychological benefits for athlete
        enhancement of self-confidence, 5-6
        minimization of stress, 5
    purpose of, 3, 29
    skill progressions in, 8
    special concerns of, 10
    speed of, 8, 52, 53
    for striking sports, 63-67
Functional testing
    definition of, 29, **102**
    drills for, 38-44
    of muscle strength, 7
    prior to beginning plyometric training, 77
    progression of, 32-38
    purpose of, 29, 30-31
    timing of, 31-32
Functional training, 29-30, **102**

G
Game-type experiences, in drills, 53, 94
Glencross, D., 23
Glenohumeral joint, 91
Glick, K.R., 25
Goal keepers, 62
Golf rehab program, 97
Golgi ligament endings, 21, **102**
Golgi-like receptors, 21, 25
Golgi-Mazzoni corpuscles, 21, 25, **102**
Golgi tendon organs (GTOs), 21-22, 76, 77, **102**
Gomgeraze, K., 81
Goodwin, G.M., 24
Grant, C., 22
Gray, G., 23, 25
Griggs, P., 24
Gymnastics, 73, 83

H
Haddad, B., 22
Hayes, K.C., 22
Healing, 4, 6. *See also* Rehabilitation
Healing time, constraints of, 4, 7-8

Heat, moist or deep, 10
Heel strike, and balance, 26
Henning, C.E., 25
High-stress sport-specific drills, 79
High volt galvanic stimulation, 6
Hip strategy (for automatic postural correction), 27, **102**
Hockey, 47
Hopping (drill), 15, 29-30, 31, 39-41
Horizontal hopping and jumping, 40-41

I
In-depth jumping and box drills, 79
Injuries
    in collision and contact sports, 47
    in combat sports, 63
    functional testing following, 32
    from maximal weight training, 22
In-place jumping, 79
Intensity of training, 79, 86, 88
International Knee Documentation Committee, 30-31
Interval throwing program, 95-96
Intrafusal muscle fibers, 21, **102**
Inverted push-ups (drill), 55, **102**
Isokinetic dynamometer, 7

J
Jackson, D.W., 32
Joint afferent discharge, 22
Joint replacement surgery, 24
Judo, 63, 67
Jump training. *See* Plyometric training
Jumping activities
    drills, 13-15, 39-41
    and injuries, 32
    and plyometric training, 73-82

K
Karate, 63
Katchajov, S., 81
Kegerreis, S., 4
Kennedy, J.C., 22, 24
Kicking, 61-62, 64-65
Kinesthetic awareness. *See* Body position and movement
Knee braces, 10
Knee flexion, 11, 75
Knee injuries, 4
Knee-jerk reflex, 21

Komi, P.V., 75, 76, 77, 81
L
Lacrosse, 47
Lead-off position, 88
Learning and motor control, 19
Ligamentomuscular reflex, 22
Loaded activities
    for collision and contact sport athletes, 51-53, 59-61
    for combat sport athletes, 64-65, 66-67, 69, 71
    definition of, 8-9, **102**
    in functional testing, 38-39
    in running, 85
Lordosis, 7
Lower extremity
    functional progressions following injury to, 48-53, 64-65
    functional testing of, 33-34, 36-38, 40
Lower-quarter plyometric training, 80-81
Lynch, M.A., 25

M
Malone, T., 4
Markolf, K.L., 25
Martial arts, 63
Matthews, P.C., 24
McCarroll, J., 4
McCloskey, D.I., 22, 24
Mechanoreceptors
    and afferent mechanoreceptor input, 23, 24, 25, 76
    articular, 20-21, 22, 25
    deep (muscle-tendon related), 20, 21-22, 76, 77
    definition of, **102**
    sensory input originating from, 19-20, 22-23
    superficial (cutaneous), 20
Medical history, 77
Medicine balls, 59
Microamperage, 6
Microtrauma, 91, **102**
Miller, J., 22
Mini-squats (drill)
    bilateral, 10-11, 33-34, **102**
    unilateral, 11-13
Mirror drills, 50
Mock combat, 64
Motor control
    and balance, 25
    definition of, **102**

and learning, 19
sensory input for, 19-22
Multiplane force delivery and acceptance, 52-53,
 59-61, 64-71, **102**
Multiple response jumps and hops, 79
Multiple teammate drill, 59-60
Muscle fibers
 elongation of, 76
 extrafusal, 21, **102**
 intrafusal, 21, **102**
 and principles of plyometric training, 74-76
 slow-twitch versus fast-twitch, 75-76
Muscle spindle, 21, 23, 24, 76, **102**
Muscle strength. *See* Strength, muscular
Myotatic stretch reflex, 73

N
Neoprene sleeves, 10
Neuromuscular coordination, 77
Neurophysiology
 balance and kinesthetic awareness, 25-27
 historical perspective on, 22-25
 motor control and learning, 19
 of plyometric training, 74-77
 sensory input for motor control, 19-22
Nociceptors, 21, **102**
Nonsupport drills
 bilateral (jumping), 13-15, 39-41
 following lower extremity injury, 50-51
 unilateral (hopping), 15, 29-30, 31, 39-41

O
One-armed spin drill and test, 38, 57-58
One-leg standing test, 78
One-on-one drills
 multiple teammate drill, 59-60
 straight-on drills, 59
Open kinetic-chain rehabilitation exercise, 19, 24-
 25, 32, 77, **102**
Orthopedic screening evaluation, 78

P
Pace (of running), 86, 87
Pacinian corpuscles, 20-21, 25, **102**
Pain, 6, 8, 9, 10
Pain killers (analgesics), 6
Paine, Russ, 31, 78
Pairing, of athletes in drills, 52, 53, 64, 70, 71
Palmer, I., 22

Participation, functional progression as bridge to,
 6, 10
Patellar tendinitis, 32
Patellofemoral reaction forces, 11
Performance
 functional testing of, 29
 and motor learning, 19
 postinjury, maximization of, 4-5
Physiology. *See* Neurophysiology
Pivoting drills, 15, 50-51
Plumer, L., 79
Plyometric training
 description of, 73-74
 guidelines for, 80-81
 principles of, 74-77
 program design for, 79-80
 program development for, 77-79
 purpose of, 73-74
Plyometrics, definition of, 73, **102**
Positioning, testing for, 30
Posture, 23, 25-27
Powell, J.W., 32
Power
 functional testing of, 40-41
 and skill, 73
Power squat testing, 78
Pre-exercise examinations, 77, 78
Preseason screening, functional testing during, 31,
 40
Pressure pain endings, 21
Proprioception, 4, 19-22, 63, **102**
Proprioceptive stretch reflex, 76-77
Protective equipment
 for collision and contact sports, 47, 51
 for combat sports, 63, 64, 65, 66, 70
Psychology of injured athletes, 4, 5-6, 31, 32
Punching, 66-67
Punching bags, 59, 67
Push-up position, modified, 34-36, 38, 53-54

Q
Quadriceps contraction, controlled eccentric, 11

R
Range of motion
 and balance, 26
 functional testing of, 33, 35, 37
 restoration of, 6-7, 8, 9, 19
Recovery time, 79-80, **102**

Reflex muscle inhibition, 6

Rehabilitation
    of collision and contact sport injuries, 47
    and functional progression program, 9-10
    functional testing during, 30-32
    of runners, 84-87
    setting goals for, 3
    of throwing-related injuries, 93-94

Rehabilitation professionals, 6

Repetitions
    of hopping and jumping (test), 40
    increasing number of, 11
    and motor control, 19
    and practice, 29
    and stress, 91-93

Resistance. *See* Activity loads; Loaded activities

Retropatellar compression, 11

Revson, A., 81

Rhomberg, 25

RightWeigh equipment, 33, 37

Riley, L.H., 24

Rope jumping, 73

Ruffini endings, 20, 25, **102-103**

Rugby, 47

Running
    by distance runners, 83, 84-87
    drills for, 15, 50-51
    injuries from, 83-84
    relationship to jumping, 73
    by sprinters, 83, 87-89

S

Safety. *See* Protective equipment

SAID (Specific Adaptions to Imposed Demands)
        principle, 3, 78, 94, **103**

Self-confidence
    definition of, **101**
    following injuries, 5-6
    and program assessment, 9, 10

SEMO drill, 43-44, **103**

Shadow boxing, 66, 71

Shadow kick-boxing, 64-65

Sherrington, C.S., 20, 22

Shock absorption, 74

Shoemaker, S.C., 25

Shoulder injuries
    and forward rolls, 58
    and throwing, 91-100

Shuttle run, 42-43, **103**

Shuttle 2001 equipment, 39, 56

Sidestep cut, 17, **103**

Side-to-side jumping, 13

Simulated game experiences, 53, 94

Single-leg hopping test, 31, 78-79

Single-leg quarter squat test, 78

Single-plane drills, **103**

Single-plane force delivery and acceptance, 52

Sit-out (wrestling position), 71, **103**

Skills
    and performance, 73
    progression of, **8**

Skoglund, S., 22

Soccer, 47, 83

Softball, 47

Sparring partners, 64

Special teams, 61

Specialty players, 61-62

Specific Adaptions to Imposed Demands (SAID)
        principle, 3, 78, 94, **103**

Speed
    increases in, 8, 52, 53
    in plyometric training, 73

Spencer, J.D., 22

Spinal injuries, and range of motion, 7

Spin drill, 71

Sport participation, 6, 10

Sport positions, testing for, 30

Sprawl (wrestling position), 71, **103**

Sprinters, 83, 87-89

Stability
    limits of, 26, **102**
    testing for, 78-79, **101**, **103**

Standing balance
    description of, 25-26
    disruption of, 26-27
    and preparation for combat sports, 63

Standing jumps, 79

Standing push-ups, 34

Static exercise programs, 4

Static restraints, **103**

Static stability testing, 78, **103**

Stepping strategy (for automatic postural
        correction), 27, **103**

Step-ups (drill), 11-13, 29, 36-38, **103**

Straight cut, 17

Straight-on drills, 59

Strength, muscular
    and balance, 26
    rehabilitation of, 4, 7, 8, 19, 93

Stress
   physical, 4, 91-93
   psychological, 5, 9
Stretch, as a muscle spindle response, 21
Stretching exercises. *See* Warm-ups
Support drills
   bilateral (mini-squats), 10-11, 33-34, 38-39, **102**
   following lower extremity injury, 49-50
   unilateral (step-ups), 11-13, 29, 36-39, **103**
Support tests
   bilateral, 33-36
   unilateral, 36-38
Sway envelope, 26
Swelling, 6, 8, 9
Symmetry
   functional testing of, 33-34, 35, 37
   of movement, 9, 41
   of muscle strength, 7
Synergistic muscle activity, 25

T
Tackling dummies, stationary and hand-held, 51, 65
Tae kwon do, 63
Take-down drills, 70-71
T-drills
   cut, 43
   definition of, **103**
   shuffle, 43
Team handball, 47
Team norms, 30, 31, 40
Team sports and comradeship, 5
Tennis elbow, 98-99
Tennis shoulder, 100
Thornton, E., 23
3-point position, 57
Throwing
   and muscle strength, 7
   and range of motion, 7
   rehabilitation for, 93-94, 95-100
   repetitive stress from, 91-93
   in simulated game situations, 94
Tibia, anterior translation of, 10-11
Time
   and duration of drills, 11, 52, 64, 66, 85-87
   recovery time, 79-80, **102**
Torque-output:body-weight ratios, 7
Track and field, 83
Transcutaneous electrical nerve stimulation, 6

Transitional drills, 56, **103**
Two-on-one drills, 60-61

U
Undamped jumps, 75, **103**
Unilateral nonsupport drills (hopping), 15, 29-30, 31, 39-41
Unilateral support activities
   definition of, **103**
   drills (step-ups), 11-13, 29, 36-39, 56-58
   tests, 36-38
Unloaded activities
   for collision and contact sport athletes, 48-51, 53-58
   for combat sport athletes, 64, 69, 71
   definition of, 8-9, **103**
Up-and-down drill, 54
Upper extremity
   ergometers for, 84
   functional progressions following injury to, 53-61, 66-67
   functional testing of, 34-36, 38
Up-position (standing) drills, 67, 69-71, **103**

V
Verhoshanski, Yuri, 73, 80, 81
Vertec equipment, 41
Vertical hopping and jumping, 41
Vertical jump assessment, 30
Volleyball, 73
Volume (of training), 79
Von Arx, F., 81

W
Walking and balance, 26
Wall rebounding drills, 56
Warm-ups, 78, **88**
Weakness. *See* Strength, muscular
Weight acceptance, 9, 53
Weight-bearing drills and tests
   bilateral support drills, 10-11, 33-34, 53-55
   and closed kinetic-chain rehabilitation exercise, 24-25, 32, 33
   timing of, 9-10
   unilateral support drills, 11-13, 29, 36-38, 56-58
Weight shifting, 9, 34, 35-36, 37
Weight training
   exercise frequency in, 79
   injuries from maximal, 22

Weight training *(continued)*
   intensity of, 79
   and muscle strength, 73
   volume of, 79
Wetherald, T., 4
Wheelbarrow drill, 55, **103**
Wheelbarrow (modified push-up) position, 34-36, 38, 53-54
Wilk, Kevin, 94
Wilt, Fred, 73

Wind-up (in throwing), 92
Wolf's Law, 4, 6, **103**
Work hardening programs, 3
Work:rest ratio, 79-80
Wrestling, 47, 63, 67, 68
Wyke, B., 22, 23

Y
Yamamoto, S.K., 3

About the Authors

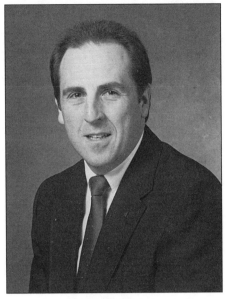

Steven R. Tippett

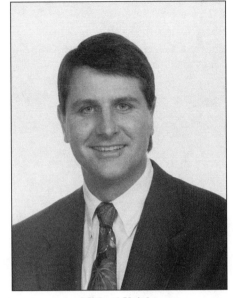

Michael Voight

Steven R. Tippett and Michael L. Voight are two of the most experienced and qualified people to write on the topic of sport rehabilitation. Both are authorities on functional progressions, having presented lectures on the topic on the national and international level.

Steve Tippett is a licensed sports physical therapist and a certified athletic trainer as well as a noted researcher, national lecturer, and sports medicine and physical therapy instructor. He is one of the original 16 sports physical therapists in the U.S. certified by the American Board of Physical Therapy Specialties.

Steve is the director of the Great Plains Sports Medicine and Rehabilitation Center in Peoria, Illinois, where he works with injured athletes, athletic trainers, and sports medicine physician specialists on a daily basis.

He is author of *Coaches Guide to Sport Rehabilitation* (Human Kinetics) and has contributed to a variety of sports medicine texts, publications, and journals. Steve is a member of the American Physical Therapy Association and the National Athletic Trainer's Association.

Michael Voight is the co-director of the Berkshire Institute of Orthopaedic and Sports Physical Therapy in Wyomissing, Pennsylvania. He is also an instructor at the University of Miami School of Medicine—Physical Therapy Division.

In addition to being a certified athletic trainer, strength coach, board-certified orthopedic therapist, and licensed sports physical therapist, Michael is a national lecturer and author of numerous articles and text chapters. Like Steve Tippett, he was one of the first 16 sports physical therapists in the U.S. certified by the American Board of Physical Therapy Specialties.

Michael is a member of the American Physical Therapy Association and the National Athletic Trainers' Association.

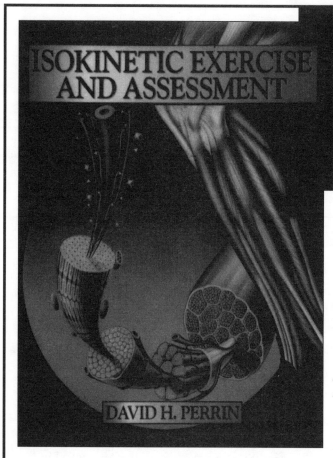